OBSTACLE RACE TRAINING

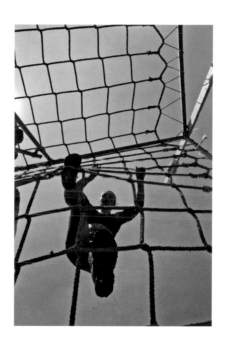

dedication

This book is dedicated to my family—a special thanks for raising me to always follow my heart and chase after dreams. It is your encouragement and unwavering support that has allowed me to always go my own way. A special thanks goes to my mother who instilled in me from a young age a love and appreciation of the woods—a love that continues to this day. She is an amazing woman in a long line of amazingly strong women who have broken boundaries and left their mark on my world.

Thank you to all who have contributed to the book: Chris Rutz, Andi Hardy, Juliana Sproles, Chris Davis and Shelley Koenig for sharing your stories; Brent Doscher of Nuvision and Jennifer Sullivan for your photos; Minna Urrey and Vanessa Runs for your editorial help. Thank you to those who have read and continue to read DirtinYourSkirt.com, supporting my endeavor as it has grown over the last couple of years.

My thanks to you, the reader, for picking up this book.

Finally, my thanks to Forest Call. This is book would not have been possible without all your help, hard work, and standing by me along the way. You are my biggest supporter, and truly the unsung hero in my life.

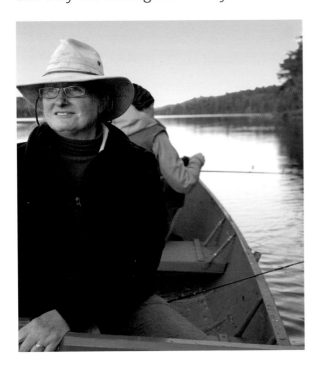

To my mother. Thanks for teaching me the virtues of nature, and giving me a lifelong love of the outdoors.

OBSTACLE RACE TRAINING

HOW TO BEAT ANY COURSE, COMPETE LIKE A CHAMPION AND CHANGE YOUR LIFE

MARGARET SCHLACHTER

With a foreword by Hobie Call

TUTTLE Publishing

Tokyo | Rutland, Vermont | Singapore

Published by Tuttle Publishing, an imprint of Periplus Editions (HK) Ltd.

www.tuttlepublishing.com

Copyright © 2014 Margaret Schlachter

Library of Congress Cataloging-in-Publication Data for this title is in progress

ISBN 978-0-8048-4391-1

Distributed by

North America, Latin America & Europe
Tuttle Publishing
364 Innovation Drive
North Clarendon, VT 05759-9436 U.S.A.
Tel: 1 (802) 773-8930
Fax: 1 (802) 773-6993
info@tuttlepublishing.com
www.tuttlepublishing.com

Japan
Tuttle Publishing
Yaekari Building, 3rd Floor
5-4-12 Osaki, Shinagawa-ku, Tokyo 141 0032
Tel: (81) 3 5437-0171
Fax: (81) 3 5437-0755
sales@tuttle.co.jp
www.tuttle.co.jp

Asia-Pacific
Berkeley Books Pte Ltd
61 Tai Seng Avenue, #02-12
Singapore 534167
Tel: (65) 6280 1330
Fax: (81) 6280 6290
inquiries@periplus.com.sg
www.periplus.com

First edition
17 16 15 14   6 5 4 3 2 1   1401TWP

Printed in Singapore

TUTTLE PUBLISHING® is a registered trademark of Tuttle Publishing, a division of Periplus Editions (HK) Ltd.

CONTENTS

Foreword

By Hobie Call

I first met Margaret Schlachter at the 2011 Spartan Death Race. She liked to study people's workout routines and philosophies in training for this new sport of Obstacle Course Racing. She was intrigued with the rock workout I used to train for the Death Race, said she had tried it a few times, and was wondering how I came up with it, why, and did I think it worked well in preparing me for such a race. I had joined the obstacle course racing world that spring and was undefeated going into the Spartan Death Race. She had watched me enter the sport and was eager to learn more about my background and training.

Margaret has a unique perspective on obstacle course racing. She raced in the very first Spartan Race, held outside of Burlington, Vermont in 2010, with only about 500 participants. She truly has been involved in the sport since its beginnings. She lived close to Joe Desena, the founder of the Spartan Race series, worked and trained with him for a couple of years, getting to know the behind-the-scenes side of the sport. She also really enjoys getting to know the elite athletes in the sport, exploring their backgrounds, how they train, their diets, the gear and shoes they choose to wear, and why. We became friends quickly after the Death Race and we often talk about training, diets and nutrition.

In the last three years, Margaret has also built up quite the racing resume herself. She has participated in almost 50 obstacle races from the Warrior Dash, to Superhero Scramble, Spartan Race, Rugged Maniac, Tough Mudder, Spartan Death Race, Worlds Toughest Mudder, Fuego y Agua Survival Run, and many more. Her experiences led her to starting a blog called DirtInYourSkirt.com, which was named the sports blog of the year by Sports Weblog for the 2012 Weblog Awards. Today she is one of the top-ranked women in the sport and enjoys sharing her knowledge with new racers. You're sure to fall in love with this sport as so many of us have, as Margaret shares the challenges, uniqueness and fun of obstacle racing.

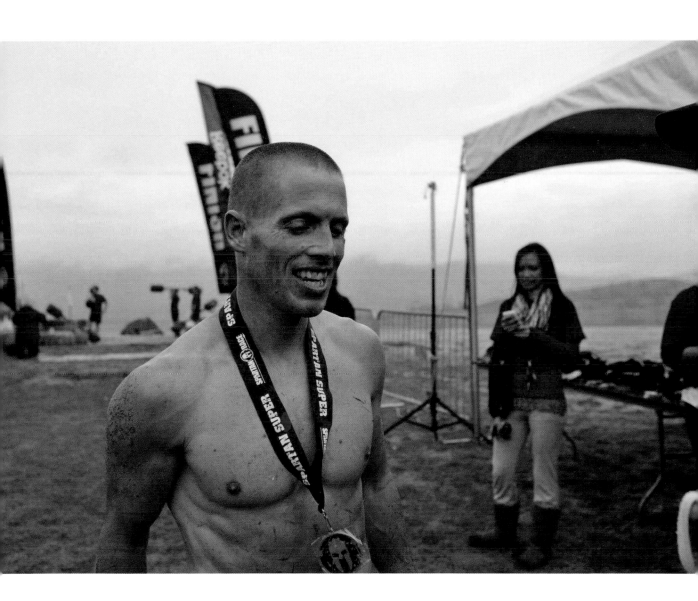

Introduction

I sat in the front seat of the police car and felt my world crumbling around me. It had only been a few weeks since I heard the news that I would not only be unemployed in a month, but I would simultaneously lose my home, having been a dorm parent the last three years. The 2008 economic downturn had taken an extra couple years to hit private education, but now I was becoming a casualty of budget cuts at Stratton Mountain School. This wasn't just the school that had employed and housed me for three years; it was also my alma mater, the same school that established a citizenship award in my honor. Since being made redundant I had numbed my emotions each night, looking down a bottle, and then hiking away the hangover each morning as penance for my actions. I

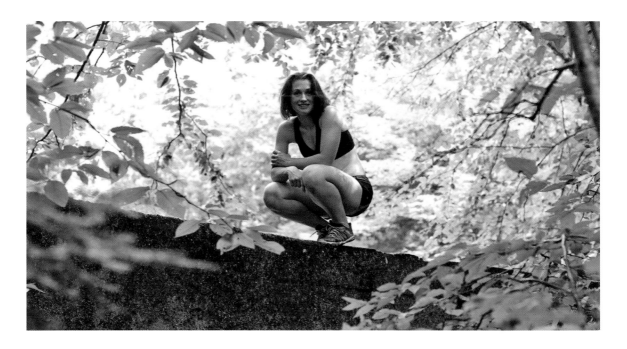

was literally spending days escaping from my problems to the only place I could think of: the woods. I was out of shape, having spent my post-college early twenties working hard and playing harder. I had packed on about 20 pounds since graduating, enjoying wing night and $2 drafts in excess. It all seemed to catch up with me that rainy night.

It was early summer 2009. I sat in that police car in the pouring rain, about to take a Breathalyzer test and most likely add another layer to my current troubles with a DUI. After I blew into the device I tested just above the legal limit, but the kind police officer took pity on me and offered me the chance to take a field sobriety test, saying, "I don't trust what these things say anyway." As I climbed out of the police car I could feel my heart ready to leap out of my chest. I carefully listened to the officer's instructions and tried to do as he said, while the two inebriated passengers in my car watched breathlessly. The rain poured down hard on me as I took the test then rejoined the officer to discuss the outcome: I had passed. I had dodged the biggest bullet of my life. It was at this moment that I knew I needed to make a change.

In fall 2009 I started a new job at a new school, holding that experience close to my chest and not revealing it to anyone. However, as I look back at that night, I know that it was my brush with disaster that started me on the journey that led me to write this book. Shaken after that period in my life I now refer to as "the black hole," I knew I could not continue to live that lifestyle, a time bomb that would eventually go off. I jumped with both feet into the new job, stopped going out so frequently, and started to look to other things in life for fulfillment. It was time to shift from one extreme to another; I just didn't know yet what it would be.

One wintery day in early 2010, I was browsing Facebook when a friend's "like" popped onto my newsfeed. It was for a new event called the Spartan Race. I felt compelled to find out what this was. I Googled it and learned it was this new sort of race called "obstacle course racing" and it would be held in May outside of Burlington, Vermont. At the time, I was living less than two hours from the race site, in central Vermont, and thought I would give it a try. I thought maybe this would be what I was looking for. I had been a two-sport varsity athlete in college and it had been years since I was in competition for myself. I spent my post-college life coaching other student athletes, but my own internal fire for competition had gone up in smoke.

The Spartan Race was advertised as a 2-mile trail run with obstacles mixed in. The ad said you would get wet and muddy, and that there would be fire. It was so new and so different that I decided to try it out. I showed up on race day not knowing that it would change the direction of my life. Over those two miles I made all the rookie mistakes. I felt like I didn't do anything right--but I knew one thing at the end: I loved it! I knew I had rediscovered something that I'd lost years ago. The spark of my inner competitor was relit, and it was time for me to regain who I was and discover who I could be. I found a few more obstacle course races that year, finishing in the top 25 percent but not breaking any records or placing anywhere near a podium. I was slow and I failed a lot, but I learned a little bit more with each race, loving it more and more. I was just out in the mud getting dirty--and experiencing something completely new.

In winter of 2011, I hesitantly signed up for an event called Tough Mudder, a 10-mile obstacle course race. Up to that point, the handful of races I'd run had all been 5Ks (about 3.1 miles) and I had never been a "runner" nor thought about running a 10-mile race. Just one month before the event I started a crash exercise program. I had coached alpine skiing for almost seven years and women's lacrosse for five years. I knew what it took to train and how to train, so I got on the trails and trudged though the miles. My longest practice run was an 8-miler just prior to race day. As I stepped up to the Tough Mudder starting line I was nervous, wondering if I would even be able to finish. As I took off on the trail, I turned my brain off and just moved. The race is a blur; all I remember is crossing the finish line and finding out I had finished third for women in my heat and in the top 25 for the day. I was told I qualified for the World's Toughest Mudder, a 24-hour championship in December.

It took me a couple of days to commit, but I thought it was a sign, and a direction I needed to follow, so I signed up for World's Toughest Mudder. That same day I created DirtinYourSkirt.com. Until then Dirt in Your Skirt was just my personal blog, a way of holding myself accountable to my training and tracking my journey up to the race. I would record workouts and feelings on the blog. Over time, people started to catch on and wanted to learn more. The blog grew.

On August 6, 2011, I took my next major step toward where I am today, taking part in the first Spartan Race Beast, the only half-marathon-distance (13.1 miles) obstacle race at the time. It was held literally in my backyard, on my training grounds of Killington, Vermont. I showed up to that race unaware of what would happen. The race began and I took off, crossing the finish line just under three hours later and placing third overall for women. This was my first official podium in the world of obstacle course racing, run on what is still arguably one of the most challenging courses. Less than a week later I would follow it up with a podium finish at the Warrior Dash in Windham, New York. This

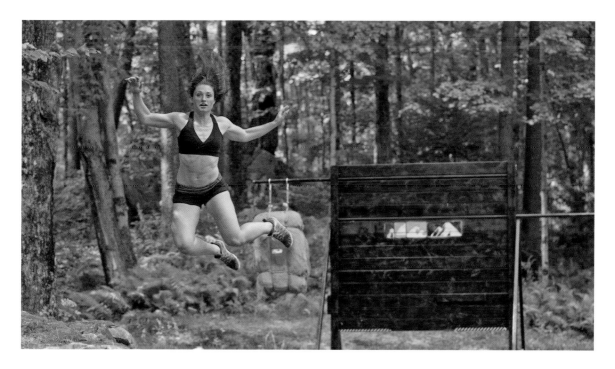

is when I knew obstacle course racing was for me. Later that year I would finish sixth in the first-ever Spartan Race World Championships held in December in Texas. The World's Toughest Mudder would not prove as successful. After 21 hours of racing, I was the last woman to drop from the race, with only two women finishing. It is certain that 2011 was the year I advanced from just being a racer in the crowd to a competitor.

With the start of the 2012 season and a second-place finish at the Spartan Race Sprint in Tuxedo, New York, a couple of companies came on board to help fund my endeavors. My racing resume grew while Dirt in Your Skirt rapidly evolved from just a hobby blog to a small business and full-blown website. At the end of the spring season, I got my first paid sponsorship. With that latest bit of encouragement, I leapt into the unknown in July 2012, quitting my daytime job in education to pursue racing full-time with the backing of sponsors and a burgeoning new business. With this single move I became the first professional female obstacle course racer, opening a new door for athletes in the sport. Throughout the 2012 season and early into the 2013 season I would pick up more podiums and more top-10 finishes. In addition to racing, I grew Dirt in Your Skirt into a forum designed to empower women to enter new sports, explore new possibilities, conquer old fears, and inspire those around them to go beyond their perceived limits. The website now features many women making differences in their own lives and the lives of those around them.

To this day I have completed close to fifty obstacle course races across the United States and internationally, of varying distances and with a variety of race organizers. Tens of thousands of users visit DirtInYourSkirt.com monthly, and we have a team of ambassadors to spread the Dirt in Your Skirt ethos: explore, conquer and inspire. I am proud to have been a part of the sport since its humble beginnings and have turned it into my vocation in life. Little did I know, sitting in a police car in summer 2009, that my brush with disaster would be the tipping point that would lead me to realize my life's passion.

I wrote this book to introduce you to all things "obstacle course racing" and "mud runs". It is designed to help you pick the right first event for you, create a training plan to get you moving, and help you to create a diet to get you going. I talk you through some of the basic obstacles you will encounter in your race, as well as how to get through race day with ease and look like a professional. I have also included personal accounts from friends who are deep into the obstacle racing world. They share their experiences and walk you through what happens after the race. Finally, we throw in plenty of insider tips and advice along the way.

Whether you do one or one hundred obstacle course races in your lifetime, you will learn something about yourself in the process and maybe, if you are like me, you will find a new passion and love. I am not going to say this book will change your life, but it just might be your tipping point.

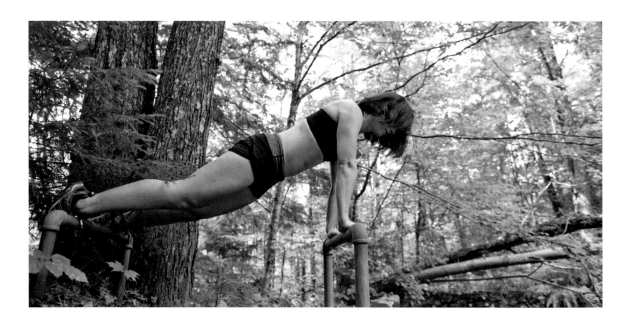

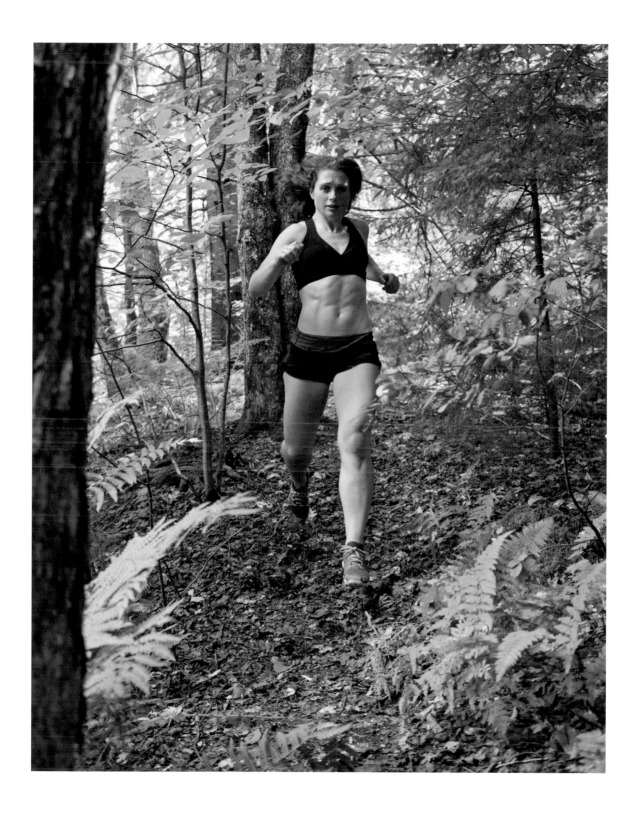

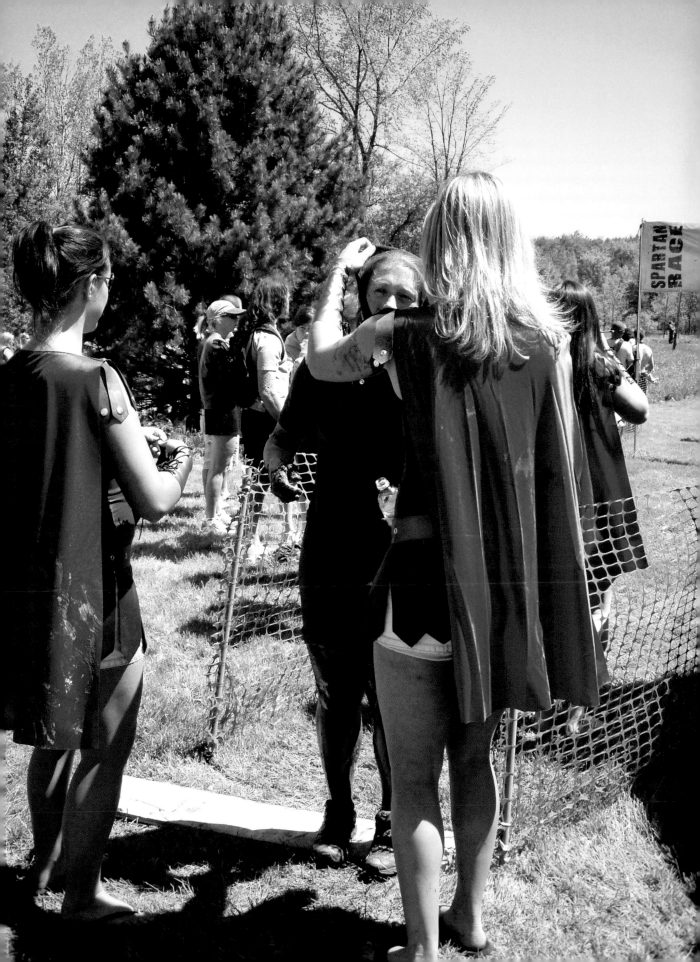

SECTION 1

INTRODUCTION TO THE SPORT

"The best way to predict the future is to create it."   —*Peter Drucker*

In spring 2010, I pulled up to the Catamount Outdoor Center outside of Burlington, Vermont and parked in a gravel lot. It was years since I had raced, and this Spartan Race would be my first-ever obstacle course race. I had no idea what to expect. As I got out of my car and looked around I saw the fire department's huge red truck and a fire blazing on the race course near the starting line. Looking in the other direction towards the finish line I saw what would be best described as an adult version of children's playground equipment. There was a wooden contraption that which you climbed up using a cargo net, then scaled down on wooden slats on the other side. What I couldn't see from my vantage point were the spear throw, 8-foot walls, barbed wire crawl, and the swimming sections that would lie ahead. It was already obvious: this was not your average race! With one slightly impulsive race entry, I began my adventure into the newly emergent worlds of mud runs[1] and obstacle course racing. I found my true passion both for sports and, ultimately, life as a professional obstacle course racer. I will be sharing those experiences as I instruct new racers on how to successfully enter this growing sport.

---

1   More about the difference between mud runs and obstacle course races in Chapter 3.

CHAPTER 1

OBSTACLE COURSE RACING EXPLAINED

Obstacle course racing immediately broke the mold when it first started in England in 1997, but it was not until 2010 that it would gain momentum in the United States. An entirely new sport was born, far outside the norm of today's conventionally organized sports. Although you may not have ever heard of it before picking up this book, obstacle course racing is one of the world's fastest growing events! Each year, hundreds of thousands of people throughout the world register and show up each weekend to race. People everywhere are opting out of the traditional 5K[2] or 10K[3] road races to venture into the world of obstacle course races. So what exactly is obstacle course racing? Time to throw out all the rule books and abandon what you thought a sport was supposed to be.

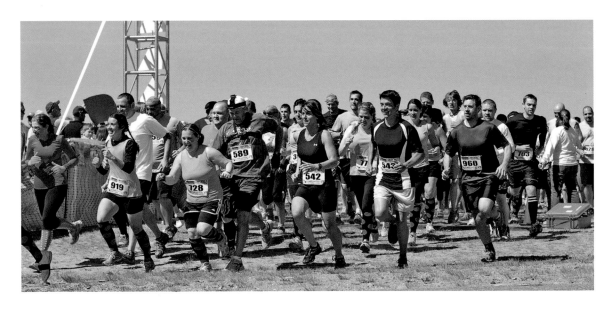

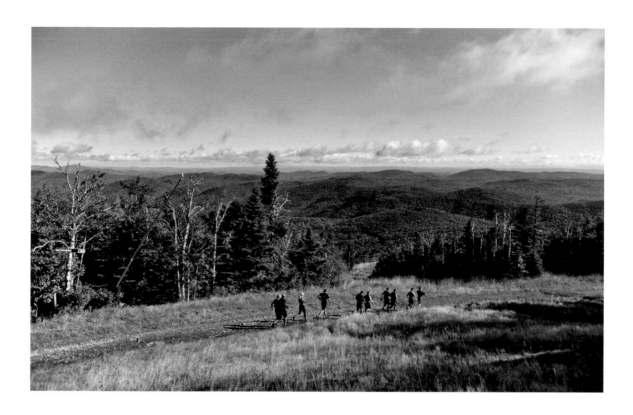

Obstacle course racing (OCR) is a sport that draws on many other sports to create a truly innovative and unique experience for the competitor. At the core of OCR you will find a running race; many racers have likened it to a combination of trail running, road running and cross-country running. Each racer travels on foot through a pre-determined course, ranging in distance from a 5K up to a marathon[4]. The terrain typically consists of trails and some dirt roads; paved roads are rarely used. Common venues for these races are ski resorts, recreational parks or other trail systems, often near larger cities. As OCR's popularity has grown, new (often smaller) regional races are emerging nationwide, helping to expand the sport at the grassroots level.

Utilizing and integrating existing terrain is one of the key features of an OCR, as the style of each race course is determined primarily by the geographical location of the race. Speaking with competitors after races, many say the most challenging obstacle was the terrain itself. Some race venues are 100 percent mountainous while others near water are almost completely flat and run on a mix of sandy beach and grass. This varying

---

4   A marathon is 26.2-mile running race. More about the distances in Chapter 3.

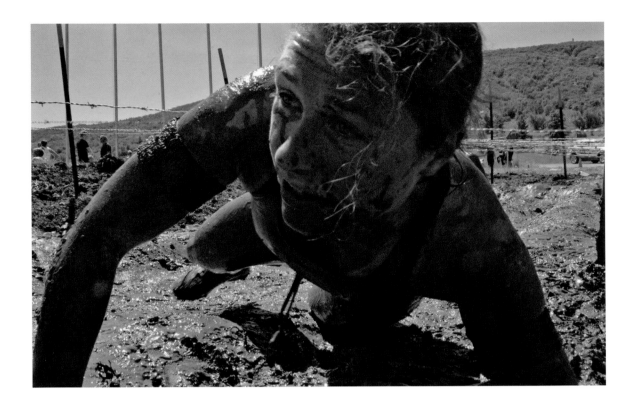

terrain can greatly affect the course layout from venue to venue and adds mystery to the competitors' experience. Some races even require bushwhacking[5] your way through the woods. One thing is guaranteed: running an OCR is not just another fun run; it's an experience and adventure!

Many OCR races not only incorporate manufactured obstacles but also utilize the specific local geographic features in their course design. It is not uncommon to encounter such obstacles as swimming across ponds, wading through mud pits, crossing streams, hiking rocky terrain, scaling downed trees, and traversing wind tunnels created by snowmaking guns. Swimming sections are never especially long or deep and, unlike other multi-sport events such as triathlons, racers complete these obstacles fully clothed and wearing shoes. You can touch the bottom of most water obstacles, and quality events are supervised by race staff or trained professionals.

One race that was particularly adept at utilizing available resources took place at a ski resort one spring, and used part of a still-frozen snowboarding half pipe as an obstacle.

---

5   "Bushwhacking" is traveling through wooded areas where there are no trails.

Yes, we climbed over the snow in May! It was the only time I've ever raced wishing I'd worn gloves. Another race held in Vermont featured a unique obstacle consisting of sticky maple syrup mixed with wood chips, called the "Shake and Bake." However, there is no question in my mind that the most memorable obstacle is the fire jump. Yes, you read that correctly; you get to jump over fire.

While the terrain is a major factor in the sport of obstacle course racing, the defining characteristics of an OCR are definitely found in the obstacles themselves[6]. A lot of the major OCR companies have designed many of their obstacles to mirror those used in military training. Specific obstacles vary from race to race, but you will normally find core obstacles such as climbing walls, barbed wire crawl[7], a heavy object pull (for example, cement blocks), carrying heavy items such as sandbags or buckets[8], running through water, scaling cargo nets and, in some races, jumping over fire or through electrified wires. Obstacles vary greatly in difficulty but racers often can choose to opt out or incur a penalty for not completing an obstacle successfully. Penalties have been known to include a set of exercises such as push-ups or burpees[9]; a time penalty can also be incurred. Obstacles can be completed individually or with the assistance of another competitor[10]. Many mud runs even encourage participants to work together and include obstacles that are virtually impossible to complete without teamwork. Each race adds in its own flavor or theme, be it gladiators with pugil sticks[11], green slime, long water slides, or other themed obstacles.

In essence, the obstacles become an equalizer, making OCR a sport not only for the elite runner. The running portion makes it a sport not just for the power-lifting champion, either. Unlike many sports that highlight only one particular athletic attribute, OCR rewards the most versatile, well-rounded athlete. It also stands apart from multi-sport events such as triathlons in which each event is performed in its entirety before moving on to the next. Obstacle course racing uniquely combines both the endurance required to traverse the course distance with the strength, speed, and dexterity to complete obstacles along the way. In any given race, a competitors might find themselves in the water, followed by a climb over an 8-foot wall, then a mile or so later more water or waist-deep mud.

---

6 Remember, this sport is called OBSTACLE course racing!
7 Sometimes it's just rope.
8 My personal favorite obstacles!
9 Burpees are explained in detail in Chapter 8.
10 I have often relied on the help of a stranger on the course, especially when scaling 10-foot (and higher) walls.
11 Remember those funny foam-tipped stick things from American Gladiators? They are used in Spartan Races!

The courses are ever-changing and obstacles are rarely in the same order from race to race, making each race a new experience. Courses are specifically designed to challenge all parts of the body, which makes OCR stand out from many other sports and allows for more creativity in training and course design. Depending on specific goals, anyone from a weekend warrior to a professional athlete can find enjoyment in pushing him or herself in an obstacle course race.

I have heard from both runners and non-runners that their first completed OCR felt like a metaphor for their lives; you may not always know what to expect, but when you encounter obstacles, you have to find a way up, over, or around it before you can continue. Many participants describe becoming "hooked" on how they feel once they complete a race and receive a finisher medal around their neck. One race company has even coined a phrase about the feeling: "You'll know at the finish line[12]" which could not be more true! For me, it is a chance to run around and feel like a kid again. Each race is like playing around on a giant adult playground.

The beauty of obstacle racing is it gives us all a chance to step outside our comfort zones and experience something real. So many of us are stuck in cubicles, trapped in an urban jungle where traffic, construction sites and sky-high buildings are the only obstacles available. Many of us live devoid of all nature, and exercise on treadmills and in warehouses. Obstacle course racing gives us all a chance to get back to nature, pound our feet on some dirt, roll in the mud, get dirty and tap into our more primal selves so we experience life raw and unedited. This is an experience long forgotten or thrown by the wayside in many sports today. This is the real reason to enter an OCR: so you can remember what it is to play and, more importantly, to LIVE.

---

12 The Spartan Race motto.

CHAPTER 2

A BRIEF HISTORY OF THE SPORT

Throughout history, people have been engaged in multi-sport events, from the first documented pentathlon in 708 B.C. to, much more recently, triathlons and adventure races. People have wanted to challenge themselves physically in more than one arena. Obstacle course racing and mud runs are the latest of these dynamic sporting events.

Although the obstacle course racing phenomenon only reached mass popularity in 2010, it had actually been around for years before then. Obstacle courses have been a staple in the armed forces for decades, used by the military as a key part of training. In 1993, Camp Pendleton (the Marine Corps base in California) organized the first World

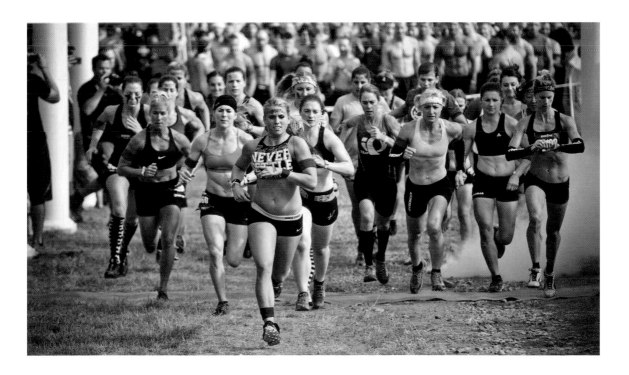

Famous Mud Run, arguably one of the first obstacle course races open to the public in the United States. It is still hosted by the Marine Corps and features both a civilian and a military category.

While the World Famous Mud Run was building ground in the United States, another event had already been around for over five years: the Tough Man Challenge. This one-day event is put on annually by Billy "Mr. Mouse" Wilson, a mad genius with a military background, on his 600-acre farm near Wolverhampton, England. It takes place at the end of January, often in freezing winter conditions, and consists of a cross-country run of 7 to 8 miles followed by an assault course. Participants report that it is tougher than any other race worldwide, featuring 25 obstacles including a slalom run up and down a hill, ditches, jumps, freezing water pools, fire pits and so on; obstacles vary slightly each year. The organizers claim that running the course involves risking barbed wire, cuts, scrapes, burns, dehydration, hypothermia, acrophobia, claustrophobia, electric shocks, sprains, twists, joint dislocation and broken bones. It is very much on the extreme end of the obstacle course racing and mud run category. This is exactly how Wilson designed it.

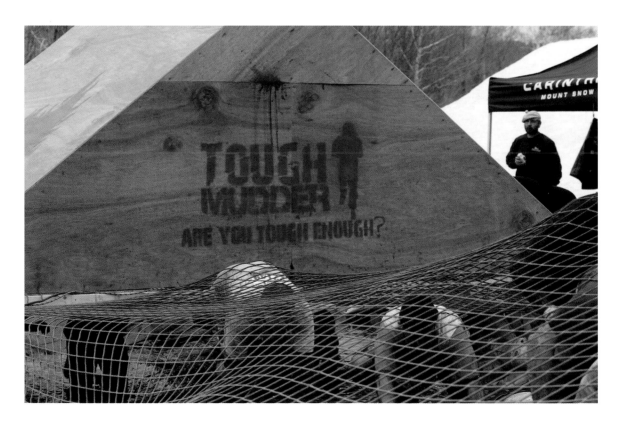

It was not until 2010 and the emergence of the "Big Three" onto the screen—the Warrior Dash, the Spartan Race and Tough Mudder—that obstacle course racing and mud runs left the military base and reached a mass audience. The first Warrior Dash actually took place a year earlier in Joliet, Illinois on July 18, 2009, as an extension of an event called the Great Urban Race. Today the Warrior Dash, created by parent company Red Frog Events, is one of the largest in the OCR sector, with a total of more than a million participants and approximately 50 events each year, each of which features the brand's iconic Viking hats and party atmosphere.

The second series, the Spartan Race, had slightly different beginnings. In 2004, former adventure racer Joe Desena and triathlete Andy Weinburg set out to put on a race like no one had seen before. It was, and still is, known as the Death Race[13]. Famous for its misdirection and absurdity, the New York Times called it "part Jackass, part Survivor[14]" in a 2010 video piece. This event grew over the years and in 2010 the two enlisted Brian Duncanson, Shaun Bain, Noel Hanna and Mike Morris, friends from Joe's adventure racing days, and former Death Racers Richard Lee and Selicia Sevigny to create a new event that was more accessible to a mass audience. In May 2010, the first Spartan Race was held outside of Burlington, Vermont. About 500 people participated in that first event, which was followed by a few more races that year in both the US and Canada. In 2011, the Spartan Race became the first race series to offer cash prizes. It is now known for the elite athletes who race competitive heats at each race as well as its appeal among the weekend warriors who want to challenge themselves. A few signatures of their events are the spear throw and course designs; former adventure racers carefully design each course. In early 2013, Spartan Race was rebranded the "Spartan Race" after the first major long-term sponsorship deal in obstacle course racing was announced. Spartan Race's aim is to turn obstacle course racing into a fully professional sport and ultimately an Olympic event.

The final Big Three member is the Tough Mudder, founded in 2010 by Englishmen Will Dean and Guy Livingstone. Dean had attended Harvard Business School and used the Tough Mudder concept in the annual Business Plan Competition. The plan was a finalist but his professors claimed it would never work in practice. Proving them wrong, Dean and Livingstone launched the first event on May 2, 2010 at Bear Creek Ski Resort near

---

13 www.YouMayDie.com is the Death Race website. It really is like no other event. They don't tell you when it starts and you don't know when it's going to end!
14 From http://www.nytimes.com/video/2009/07/06/sports/1194841322337/surviving-the-death-race.html

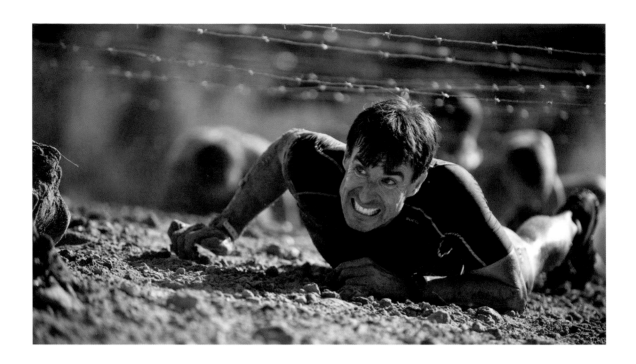

Allentown, PA. The event had 4,500 participants. They would go on to have 14 events in 2011 and 28 events in 2012, and now boasts the most participants of any mud run or obstacle race series annually across a handful of countries. The Tough Mudder philosophy was to create a series to test toughness, fitness, strength, stamina and mental grit all in one place and all in one day.

According to Tough Mudder's website (toughmudder.com), "FACT — Marathon running is simply boring. And the only thing more boring than doing a marathon is watching a marathon. Road running may give you a healthy set of lungs, but will leave you with as much upper body strength as Keira Knightley. At Tough Mudder, we want to test your all-around mettle, not just your ability to run in a straight line, on your own, for hours on end, getting bored out of your mind."

There is no doubt that, as obstacle course racing continues to grow and evolve, other events will come in and continue to help shape and evolve the sport of the future. With the explosion of shows like *American Ninja Warrior* and other obstacle-based shows it is just a matter of time before obstacle course racing finds itself on major network television and beyond. The future is bright for this sport racing and, with millions each year competing, it is destined to continue to grow.

CHAPTER 3

TYPES OF RACES AND RUNS

I f you were to talk to a hundred people in the obstacle racing world, a hundred different descriptions might might be given about the sport. As the genre has grown over the past couple of years, many monikers have been given to these individual events: Mud Runs, Mud Dashes, Fun Runs, Obstacle Course Races, Challenges, Rucks, MOBs[15] and so on. Really, all events can be split up into two main categories: mud runs and obstacle course

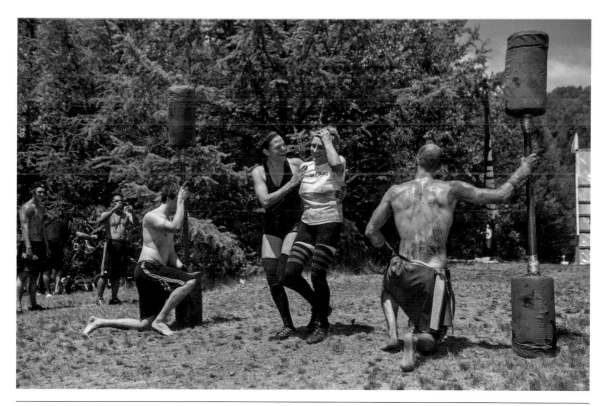

15 MOB is a term coined by Active.com to refer to all mud runs and obstacle races. It is not a commonly used term. However, as active.com is the leading online registration website, it's important to recognize the name.

races. Both feature many of the same elements and sometimes even the same obstacles. Both often hand out finisher medals or prizes to those who complete the course, and both often feature mud as their signature element. The difference lie in how the race is run for example, some types of races are timed, other aren't. There are several ways to determine whether an event is a mud run or an obstacle course race.

Mud Runs

The first tell-tale sign of a mud run is the name of the event. Often an event's name itself gives away its intentions. Events that include "challenge," "mud run," "dash," "fun," or "playground" in their names normally indicate that the event is indeed a mud run and not a race per se, and often tout themselves on their websites as such. Mud runs often focus on teamwork and camaraderie with other participants, often including obstacles that clearly require teamwork to complete, thereby taking the individual out of the equation.

Mud runs are often equated with easier events that encourage costumes and dressing up. This may be true in many of the shorter and smaller events, but as more and more events flood the market, mud runs too have come to include a diversity of offerings, appealing to a wide variety of participants. While some focus on the costumes and come to include team names, many organizers are now building out mud runs that are truly challenging and emphasize teamwork and physical ability, without a clock timing the performance of an individual participant. This option has become very appealing to many as they look to enter the world of obstacle courses.

The most famous of all the mud runs is easily Tough Mudder. Tough Mudder is a 10 to 12 mile mud run featuring impressive obstacles; one of its signatures is called "electro-shock therapy," in which participants run through a series of live electrical wires. Tough Mudder is also known for obstacles requiring competitors' mutual help to complete, such as 10-foot walls, and an obstacle resembling a skate quarter pipe that participants must run up. Tough Mudder, generally considered one of the originals in the sport (one of the "Big Three"), has carved a unique niche for itself. Founders have built their company as a "challenge, not a race."[16] Tough Mudder starts each wave of participants by reciting the same pledge:

---

16 With the exception of World's Toughest Mudder, a 24-hour obstacle course race held annually by Tough Mudder.

As a Tough Mudder I pledge that:
- *I understand that Tough Mudder is not a race but a challenge.*
- *I put teamwork and camaraderie before my course time.*
- *I do not whine - kids whine.*
- *I help my fellow Mudders complete the course.*
- *I overcome all fears.*[17]

Tough Mudder is the most challenging mud run and holds events all over the world, with upwards of 10,000 or more participants in a single weekend. Tough Mudder is an event that will challenge the most hardened athlete or weekend warrior.

There are many smaller events, such as Hardcore Mudd Run, that are taking their cues from Tough Mudder, setting up mud runs that are shorter in distance but still offer challenging obstacles that appeal to all fitness levels. As the category continues to grow, more and more smaller, regional events will enter the market.

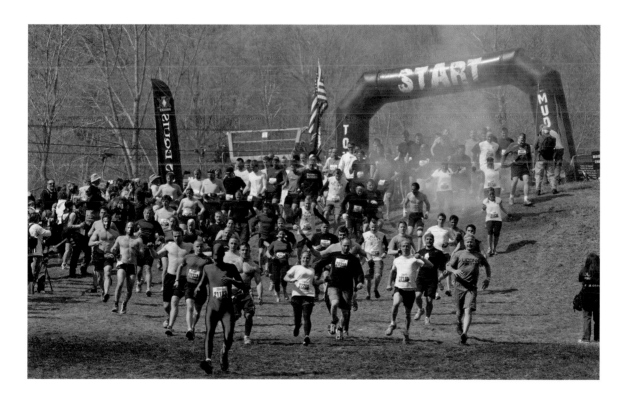

---

17 From http://toughmudder.com/history-of-tough-mudder/

Obstacle Course Races

People love to compete, and we love to race and judge ourselves against our peers. For centuries humans have competed on a variety of battlefields, from a Roman Coliseum to a farmer's field or, more recently, in conference rooms all over the world. In addition to competing, we like to like to have an objective tool with which to gauge themselves; hence the advent of many time-based sports in our modern day OCR.

On the surface, obstacle course racing and mud runs appear very similar, as they both involve a trail-based run and a wide array of obstacles. The largest difference between the two is the presence of a clock (or more commonly, a chip-based timing system) in OCR. At the end of an OCR there are awards for top overall finishers, and sometimes age group awards as well. If there is some doubt as to whether an event is a mud run or an obstacle course race, the presence of the word "race" in the name or first couple sentences of its description, or of an award ceremony, are key tip-offs as to the intentions of the event. Spartan Race is at the forefront of the serious obstacle course races.

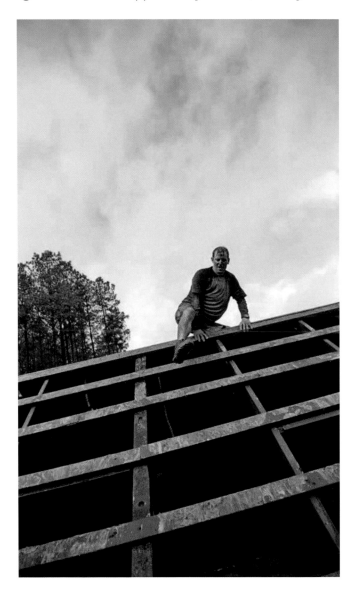

There are a few other indicators that an event is a race and not a mud run. One is the presence of an early morning "competitive" or "elite" heat. As obstacle course racing establishes itself as a sport, more and more race organizers are establishing these heats to allow all the competitive athletes to race one another at once (much like the elite runners in the Boston Marathon who take off before the masses). It is in these heats that the full-time obstacle racers are emerging. Winners may even receive prize money. In the case of Spartan Race, this is the heat from which the top athletes are ranked worldwide. Spartan Race and, more recently, the Superhero Scramble both offer cash prizes to top finishers, pushing obstacle course racing to the professional level. Prizes in these races can range from a few hundred dollars to a few thousand dollars for the winner. Both Tough Mudder and Spartan Race host world championship races where the winner can take home purses worth tens of thousands of dollars.

Another tip-off is the presence of penalties for failed obstacles. Different race organizers have different penalties for failed or skipped obstacles: for Superhero Scramble it's dizzying spins with your head on the butt of a baseball bat, whereas Spartan Race has the athletes complete a set of 30 infamous burpees[18]. At the original Spartan Race in 2010, the penalty was push-ups. Other race organizers have used time penalties, and some organizers such as Norway's Viking Race have even discussed requiring additional running. Either way, in a race be prepared to do a little bit extra if you can't make it up, over, through or under an obstacle.

By no means do you have to be an elite or competitive athlete to complete an obstacle course race. **Everyone can complete an obstacle course race.** Many people have the impression that you have to have huge muscles and be an elite athlete to even try. On the course there are people of all shapes and sizes, everyone from your weekend warrior, couch potato, CrossFit athlete, road runners, lean trail runners, former collegiate athletes, to truly elite athletes. In 2012, the Spartan Race points world champion Cody Moat also won the USATF[19] Trail Marathon and 50-miler Nationals, showing that there isn't one type of person or body that makes you good at obstacle course racing. Don't let words like "elite" or "competitive" scare you away. The majority of the people who race are weekend warriors, just looking to get out and try something new, and drawn to the idea of knowing how they stack up against the competition. This is the attitude of over 90 percent of the people racing. Race organizers have "open heats" designated throughout the day for the majority to race in. All of these open heats are timed using electronic chips, and results show how competitors finish in their specific heat, in their gender, in their age group,

---

18 You will be hearing a lot more about burpees in the upcoming chapters!
19 USATF—USA Track & Field, the governing body of track and field events.

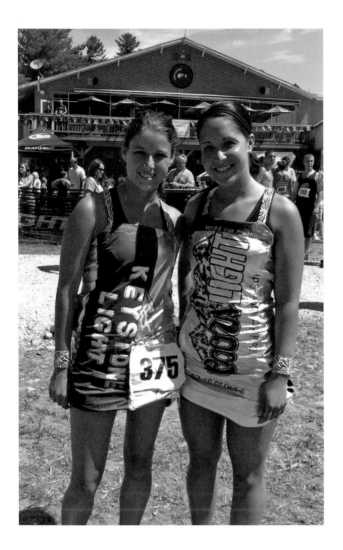

and overall. Results are presented in similar fashion to the results of, say, the Boston Marathon.

The difference between the "open" and "competitive" heats has to do with the prizes and the enforcement of penalties. Racers in the competitive heats are held strictly to the completion of obstacles and to the correct form on any penalty exercises. In many competitive heats, athletes are not able to receive outside assistance from staff or other personnel and, in some cases, are not allowed to receive help from other competitors to complete an obstacle. However, in the open heats, the rules are less rigid and racers are allowed to receive help from personnel and are encouraged to help each other to complete obstacles. In many open race situations, racers are even allowed to modify the penalty exercise if they are unable to complete the strict version. I have personally seen more variations of the burpee in my years of racing than any other exercise in decades of athletics! The open heats allow you to compete at your best and to push yourself. It is strongly recommended that you start an obstacle race series in an open heat. Although, anyone can sign up for a "competitive heat" if they really want to challenge themselves, normally for an additional registration fee.

As with everything in life, there is one major exception in obstacle course racing: Warrior Dash is one of the largest organizations in the sport (along with Spartan Race, Tough Mudder, followed by Superhero Scramble, Rugged Maniac, Ruckus, and other smaller events) and breaks all the rules stated in this chapter about what a "race" is. There are no specially designated "competitive" or "open" heats; in any given heat, you race against every other person at all ability levels. Once all heats have been completed, the fastest competitors of the day receive awards both overall and in their age group. There is also no penalty for failed obstacles, which distinguishes it from other organizers putting on races. The Warrior Dash race is primarily a 5K obstacle course race geared towards the new or casual racer, while still allowing people to see where they stack up. You have the choice of showing up on race day and just having a good time, or going for a personal best. Warrior Dash is known for the festival/party atmosphere after the race and appeals to a wide variety of competitors, leading it to be known in some circles as the "gateway" obstacle course race.[20]

Whichever kind of event you are looking for, be it a mud run or obstacle course race, there is great fun to be had. The choice depends on your preferences and the level of intensity you are looking for. For the sake of simplicity, I refer to both categories of runs throughout the rest of the book simply as "obstacle course races" or OCR, although as stated in this chapter there is a slight difference. The one thing that I have learned after 50 or so races is that, while these categories provide a general guide, each individual event organizer is slightly different, so it's important to check out a bunch and find the one that suits your needs and your personality.

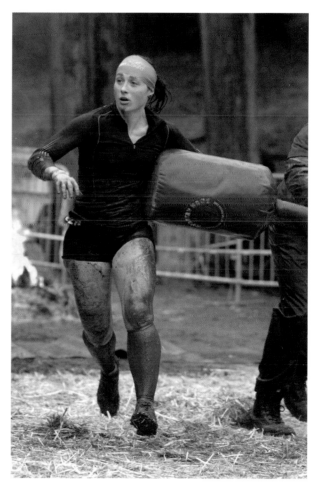

---

20 In 2013 Warrior Dash expanded its brand from the "gateway" race to also include an Urban Race and a longer distance, 13 to 15-mile "Iron Warrior Dash".

WHERE TO START

In 2010, when my fascination with obstacle course racing and mud runs began, there were few organizations out there to pick from. It was primarily the "Big Three": Spartan Race, Warrior Dash and Tough Mudder. The first two were both 5K distance races and Tough Mudder was the longer 8 to 10-mile challenge. This basically eliminated any question of "which race," as I was just looking for races in my area.

When I began racing I was not a runner and couldn't imagine running more than a few miles. I spent the first year just having fun trying to finish the races. My second year I got the obstacle course racing bug, and got it hard. I found every race I could within a reasonable traveling distance and tried them all. I primarily still raced 5 to 6K distances but included a few longer ones. At this point I had the courage to try a Tough Mudder, tackling a distance I never thought was achievable the year before. I not only finished, but my time qualified me for the World's Toughest Mudder, a 24-hour obstacle course race. I spent the next eight months preparing for the event, in the process competing in the first-ever Spartan Race Beast, which was the first half-marathon obstacle course race. A personal highlight of 2011 was completing my first ultra-marathon, the Vermont 50, a 50K race in preparation for World's Toughest Mudder. When I stepped over the finish line of the Vermont 50, it was the first time I realized I could accomplish anything. A couple months later I would go on to tackle the World's Toughest Mudder, the most challenging race of my life. I battled beyond my limits and dug deeper than I had ever gone. In the end, I did not finish and succumbed to hypothermia 21 hours into the race; however, I completed almost 40 miles of racing overall.

It was following a comfortable racing progression that led me to a 24-hour race and an ultra marathon. The first year I spent racing the 5Ks was essential to overall growth and love for the sport. I know today that if I had jumped head-first into one of the longer events, I probably wouldn't have the passion for OCR that I do now. It's truly about picking the right race for you and your fitness level; we all want to be challenged, but first create a goal that is attainable and then build off of it to reach your dream goals. Each year I plan out my race schedule and pick a mix of races I know I can excel at, to these I add a couple that are reaches and that I know I might not finish. Each time I try a new race or a new challenge, it helps me unlock a little bit more of my potential.

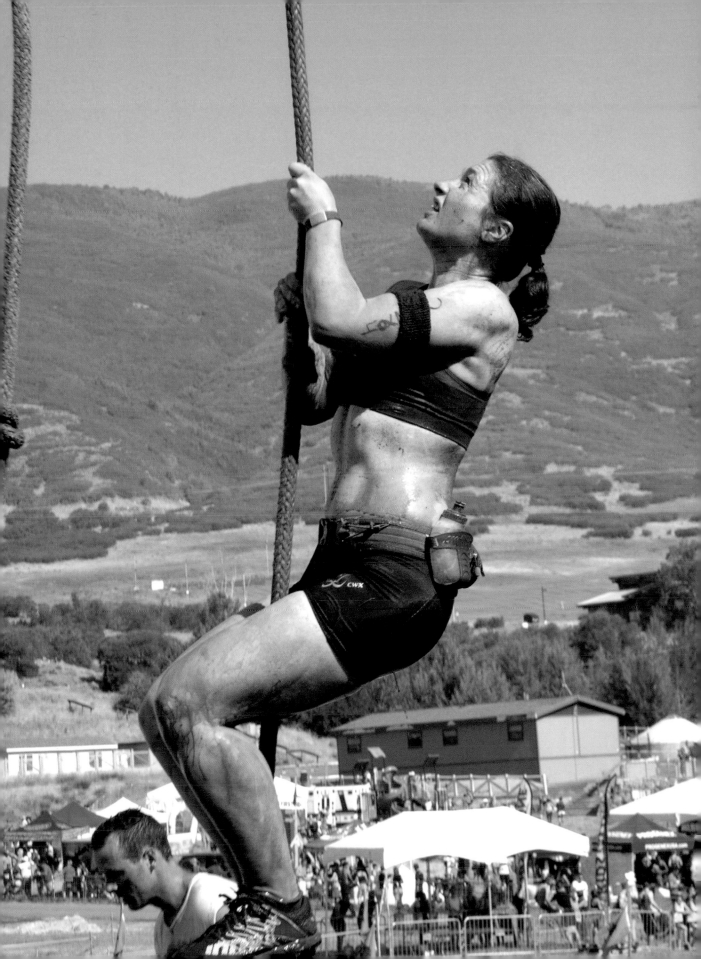

CHAPTER 4
CHOOSING THE RIGHT RACE

Obstacle course racing is the fastest growing sport in the country. Each day, more and more races are added around the country and the world. Obstacle course racing has become so popular that the popular registration website, Active.com, has recently given these races their own category: "MOB." Now you can look up 5Ks, half-marathons, triathlons, and MOBs online. The sport has even been featured in ESPN blogs and commercials. In this explosive sport, it can be daunting to wade through the sea of races to find the best one for your first experience in obstacle course racing. This book is here to help you make the right choice and make your first event memorable.

The first thing you need to do when choosing a race is decide how far you are willing to travel. As with many other sports, obstacle course racing has a few geographic hotspots around the country. If you are lucky enough to be located in the Northeastern US, Florida, South Carolina, Colorado, Texas, or California, races seems to be popping up everywhere. If you are located in Kansas, Montana, Wyoming or Utah, you will most likely be traveling a little bit farther to get to your first race. If you live in a geographic region not known for obstacle course racing, check the closest major city; chances are you will find at least one obstacle course race. Just because you don't live in a current hotbed of obstacle course racing doesn't mean that you won't find a race, because more and more events flood into this category every week. It is probably only a matter of time before a race is in your backyard.

Once you have located races in an accessible area, the second thing you want to consider is whether you are looking for an obstacle course race or a mud run. As discussed in Chapter 3, there are differences between a race and a mud run. If you are just looking to get out there and try something new, then a mud run may appeal to you. Because they're not timed (which can take the pressure off and allow the event to be more fun), many people find mud runs to be more low-key; these events often do not have penalties for failed obstacles or offer the option to opt out if an obstacle is too challenging. Mud runs can be the perfect type of event if you have a group of friends of varying fitness levels who want to accomplish the event together.

For those people with competitive juices flowing through their veins, an obstacle course race will be the event of choice. These events time you with an electronic chip and rank you at the end of the race. They tend to be a bit more serious. People are more competitive, but still willing to help out other racers. Obstacle course races often have a penalty if you fail to complete an obstacle; in Spartan Race it is the infamous 30 burpee requirement, while in the Superhero Scramble it is a dizzying bat spin. Other race organizers employ push-ups, alternative running loops, or other penalties.

Having completed over 50 obstacle course races and mud runs, I know my personal preference is to race; it's the competitor in me. I like to be timed and know where I stand at the end of a race. However, this has not deterred me from the occasional mud run. Mud runs are just as fun and can be (depending on the race organizer) just as challenging. No matter what type of event you pick as your first experience, you will be happy at the end of the race, having accomplished something new.

Now that you know where you plan to go and what type of event you want to do, you can decide the length of the race. If you are lucky, you will be able to pick between a couple different race organizers. The choice of distance and the race organizer can make all the difference in your experience. With the massive growth of the sport, event distances now range from short mile-long dashes to ultra-marathon and 24-hour long events. It can be overwhelming at times to look at all the different races and the different distances available.

The secret to a successful first race is to pick a distance you can handle. It may sound most impressive to talk with friends about how your first obstacle course race or mud run was over ten miles long, but the reality is if your body is not ready for that sort of distance you will find yourself miserable come race day. The best thing to do is start off with a shorter race or mud run; the ideal distance for your first race is a 5K to 10K. The majority of events fall in this 3 to 6-mile range. You may have run marathons and half-marathons before, but an obstacle course race will zap the energy from even the toughest athlete in ways you can't imagine.

During one race, I ran a couple miles with an excellent ultra marathoner I had met the year before during the Vermont 50. As I ran with Amy, we chatted; she was running the one-loop option for the race while I was running two loops.[21] We talked about the course and I asked her what she thought so far about her first obstacle racing experience. She said, "This is really fun, but this is REALLY hard!" She told me she planned to stick to trail

---

21 Many races offer a longer, more challenging race option for elite runners by requiring participants to circle the same course twice!

running thereafter. The next weekend she won a challenging 50-mile ultra-marathon. The Spartan Race Vermont Beast she had just run is arguably the hardest obstacle course race in the country, and she ran it as her first race; it is one of the longest races (one loop equals 15 miles) and one of the most mountainous. Without a crystal ball, it is hard to predict what Amy might have said had she raced a shorter or less challenging race for her first event, but it shows that even if you are comfortable running the distance, when you add obstacles into a race it is a completely different thing.

Finally, once you have decided on a comfortable distance to tackle, the last thing you need to do is pick the race itself. In terms of timing, it is best to give yourself one to two months to train for a race. The final factor is the race organizer. If you live in a place where the races are numerous, you will have a lot of options; other regions may not present many options and you may have only one race nearby. Before clicking the final "register" button on your chosen race's website, you should visit the websites and Facebook pages of all race options available to you. In this digital age you can easily find information about these events; most have a website and a Facebook page, which is open to the public and can be found with a simple internet search. A quick YouTube search can also give you insight to a specific course, if the organizer has run an event there in the past. Many people make their own videos using a point of view camera. These can give you an opportunity to see what the event will be like before signing up. With so many new races popping up, the available experiences are often varied. A few minutes of research online can play a major role in finding the right race.

I love the small homegrown events, and the professional racing community views them as an important part of the sport as a whole. Be aware, though, that in these smaller, local races the obstacles typically tend to be smaller, and the post-race festival areas not as exciting. It is best to find an event where the company has run a few races and worked out the logistical kinks that come along with registration, parking, and obstacles typically. If you are lucky enough to have a Warrior Dash, Reebok Spartan Race, Superhero Scramble, Rugged Maniac, Ruckus, Merrell Down and Dirty or another of the most established race organizers near you, these are the best events to look to. Warrior, Spartan, Superhero, Rugged, Ruckus, and Merrell have all been around for years and have spent the time and money to work out all of the kinks. Normally, these race organizers have a speedy registration process, ample parking, and a great post-race festival with food, live music, games and retailers. Whether you pick a large company or a small local race, you will have fun; just remember to arrive early on race day and stay away from cotton clothing, as this book will explain later on.

Ultimately, whatever event you decide—race or mud run, 5K or half-marathon, big race organizer or small local race—your racing experience will be what you make it. I have had fun at what some have called the "lame" mud runs and have had some awful experiences with some of the most established races. It all comes down to your mind-set, your level of preparedness, and your ability to not take yourself too seriously and just have fun. In the end we all end up muddy, a little bruised, and with a great story, whether it took us a half-hour or half a day to cross the finish line. It's the experience that makes it fun!

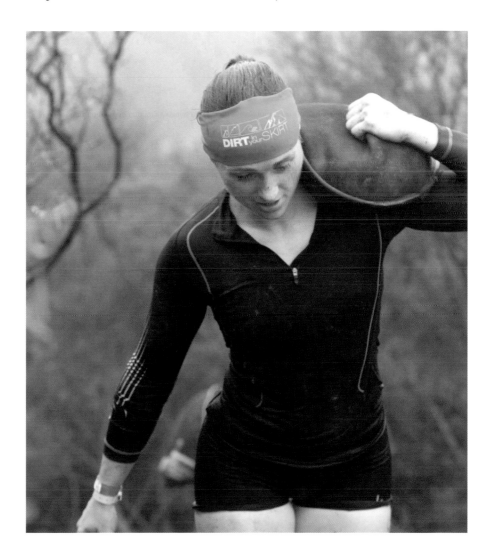

CHAPTER 5

STARTING A TRAINING PROGRAM AND CREATING A BALANCED TRAINING PLAN

As a young athlete, the phrases "failing to prepare is preparing to fail" and "train like you race; race like you train" were commonly said to me and taken close to heart. But it wasn't until I began obstacle course racing that I really knew what they meant. By this part of the book, we have reached the point where you have made the commitment to run and signed up for an event; now you are looking to put in the time to truly prepare for race day. It's time to train!

Starting A Training Program

The first thing you need to do before starting a new training program is get checked out by a doctor. It's important to make sure you do not have any limitations or that you know what those limitations are before entering into a new workout routine. Once you are checked out you know what you can or can't do. It's the important first step that many fail to take, jumping into a new training program only to find themselves derailed a few months later when an ailment suddenly arises.

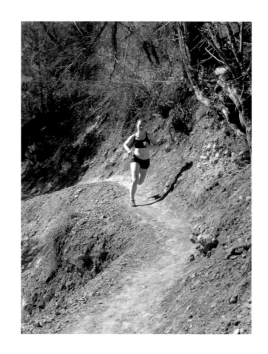

The second most important thing is to start slowly and ease into the process. It's hard to walk into a gym and see the people lifting extreme weights or sprinting past you on the trail. Training, in many ways, is like building a house:

you have to build a strong foundation in your training program first. It is the fundamental skills and early weeks of training that are critical to your overall success in any program. It's the hardest thing to do: we go into a new exercise routine with a renewed vigor and want to jump in with both feet and do it all! Unfortunately, this attitude and behavior often leads to over-exercising, overtraining, burnout and sometimes injury. Even in my own training, when learning a new skill I have to hold myself back and remember: you have to crawl before you can walk, and walk before you can run. Finally, remember that your training is always a work in progress.

Creating A Balanced Training Plan

Physical fitness is the ability to perform recreational, job-related and other daily activities successfully and without becoming overly fatigued. Ultimately, there are five elements to physical fitness:

- **Cardiorespiratory Endurance:** how the heart, lungs, and circulatory system send nutrients and oxygen to the muscles as they work
- **Muscle Strength:** how much force a particular muscle or muscle group can produce
- **Muscle Endurance:** how long the muscle or group can maintain use for an extended period of time
- **Flexibility:** how far a joint can extend in its full range of motion
- **Body Composition:** the amount of lean and fat mass that makes up your body weight

All of these things together contribute to your overall fitness level.

OCR is a unique sport in that it includes speed, endurance, coordination, agility and strength. Many popular sports today focus on one or two unique aspects, but not the complete combination. The obstacle course racer must be a fast runner, agile, strong, flexible, and adaptable. Basically, the obstacle course racer needs to have all-around fitness, also known as functional fitness. Not there yet? That's okay; many people of all fitness levels are taking on OCR, from the 400-pound man trying to improve his overall health to the former collegiate athlete looking to compete again in the post-college sporting world. This is the beauty of the sport!

This book has laid out a foundational program to help absolute beginners start to get themselves into shape and ready for their first obstacle race. This 30-day program is meant to be easy to follow and achievable for athletes of all abilities, but can be built upon and adapted as you become stronger.

Fundamentally, all obstacle course races have one thing in common: running. While many people focus on the obstacles in the race (the fun part), the main element of any good obstacle racer's training program is running. That's the workhorse of any obstacle racing training program. The specific type of running to focus on is trail running, including mountains if possible. Many think of the Kenyans and their sub-5-minute marathon miles when they hear about running, but these workouts are not like that. In fact many trail runs often include some fast walking or hiking; that is OK. It is about getting out and putting in the time on your feet.

This program focuses on the quality of the workout, not the speed. For many, the workouts will have a lot of walking in them, while others will have you running the whole time. The most important thing is to start at your own level and build from there. Each of us has our own starting point and each of us will have own challenges. The key is to do your best and build your own foundation. Most of the exercises in this program use your own body weight to provide the right resistance, helping your build the foundation that's right for you.

Four-Week Obstacle Racing Jump Start Training Program

The following is a sample training program to help you to kick-start your training. It is meant to serve a planning guide; the intensity and distances and should be modified to suit your own fitness level. One you've determined your best starting level, you can use this sample as a template for drafting your own program.

This plan uses minimal equipment and most of it can be done outside in the wilderness, on your local track or at any reasonably-sized playground. If you do not have a track near you, you can always train on the road and modify. Many of the exercises have a large number of reps in these workouts; you can break them up into sets instead of completing all the reps at once. If you're new to these moves, the techniques are illustrated just a few pages away.

All the runs are based on time rather than distance; that way, as you progress, you can still do the same workout at a higher intensity. It is important to have a schedule for yourself and your training. If you don't schedule your workouts, it's really hard to keep up with them!

Week 1:

MONDAY: Run+ Workout - 30 minute walk/jog
 Every 15 minutes stop running and complete before running again:
 10 burpees,
 10 push-ups
 10 sit-ups

TUESDAY: 30-minute jog/walk then 500 Workout
 100 sit-ups
 100 body weight squats
 100 push-ups
 100 lunges
 100 cherry pickers

WEDNESDAY: Speed Workout
 Warm-up with two laps or ½ mile warm-up
 Workout: 4 laps on track or 1 mile
 Jog the turns of the track and sprint straight aways. Complete all four laps In a row.

THURSDAY: Hike Day
 1-hour hike or incline treadmill 20lb sandbag, or other object
 (The goal is to carry extra weight and an uncomfortable object.)

FRIDAY: Rest Day

SATURDAY: Long Run or Hike Day
 1-3 hour long run or hike.

SUNDAY: Rest Day

Week 2:

MONDAY: Run+ Workout - 45 minute walk/jog
 Every15 minutes stop running and complete before running again:
 10 burpees,
 10 push-ups
 10 sit-ups

Tuesday: Rock Workout – pick a reasonable weight rock or sandbag (20 to 40lbs)

½ mile to 1- mile warm-up

Throw rock 10 times

50 squats with rock or sandbag

50 presses with the rock or sandbag above your head

50 lunges with rock or sandbag

Jog ¼ - ½ mile

Repeat 5 times

Wednesday: Speed Workout:

Warm-up with a ½ mile to mile jog and stretch

Telephone Pole Sprints: 15 min w/u then alternate sprinting and jogging in-between telephone poles for 30 minutes

Thursday: 30-minute jog/walk then 500 Workout

100 sit-ups

100 air squats

100 push-ups

100 lunges

100 pull-ups

Friday: Rest Day

Saturday: Long Run or Hike Day

1-3 hour long run or hike.

Sunday: Rest Day

Week 3:

Monday: Run+ Workout – 1 hour walk/jog

Every15 minutes stop running and complete before running again:

15 burpees,

15 push-ups

15 sit-ups

TUESDAY: 30-minute jog/walk then 800 Workout
   200 sit-ups
   150 push-ups
   200 body weight squats
   150 lunges
   100 pull-ups

WEDNESDAY: Speed Workout
   Warm-up ½ jog
   Timed 1-Mile Run – All Out
   4 rounds 100-meter sprints (30 sec rest)
   6 rounds 40-meter sprint (20 sec rest)

THURSDAY: 50's Workout
   1- mile warm-up
   50 lunges
   50 squats with sandbag or rock
   50 cherry pickers
   50 broad jumps
   50 side-to-side hops
   50 push-ups
   50 dips
   5 100-Meter Sprints

FRIDAY: Rest Day

SATURDAY: Long Run or Hike Day with added weight
   2 to 4 hour-long run or hike with sandbag, rock or other object

SUNDAY: Jog/Run – 1 hour

Week 4:
Monday: Rest Day

Tuesday: 1.5 hour walk/jog – 15 minutes – 15 burpees, 15 push-ups, 15 sit-ups

Wednesday: Speed Workout
    Warm-up with two laps or ½ mile warm-up
    Workout: 4 laps on track or 1 mile
    Jog the turns of the track and sprint straight aways. Complete all four laps in a row.

Thursday: Dirt in Your Skirt 100 Workout
    Between each exercise run ¼ -1/2 mile
    100 Side bends
    100 Burpees
    100 Pull-ups
    100 Box Jumps
    100 Wall Balls
    100 Jumping jacks
    100 Side-kicks
    100 Body Weight Squats
    100 Step-ups
    100 Sit-ups

Friday: Rest Day

Saturday: Long Run or Hike
    2 to 4 Hours

Sunday: Run 1 to 2 hours

While completing the 4-week program it is essential to listen to your body, so make sure to rest and to sleep when you need to. Sleep is as much part of your training program as the actual workout. It is during the sleep cycles that the body recovers and heals itself so you can get out there day after day.

How To

PUSH-UPS

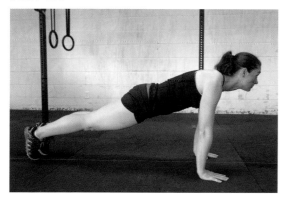 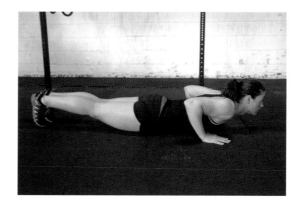

BODY WEIGHT SQUATS

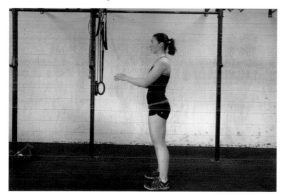 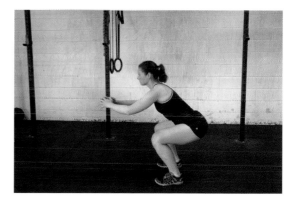

LUNGES

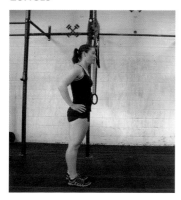 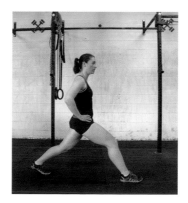 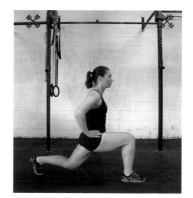

Cherry Pickers

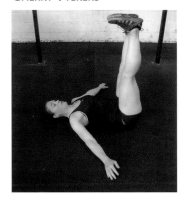 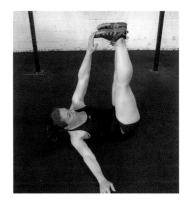 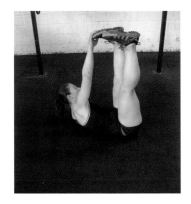

Squat with Sandbag

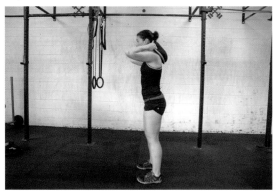 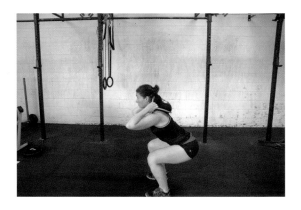

Press with Sandbag

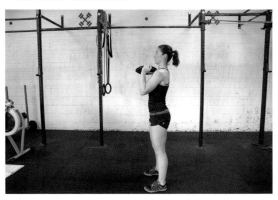 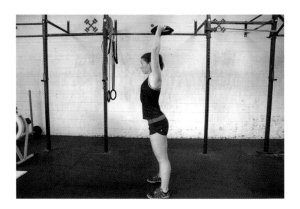

JUMPING PULL-UP

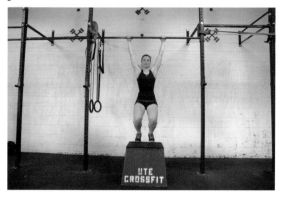 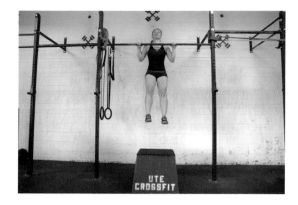

BAND PULL-UPS

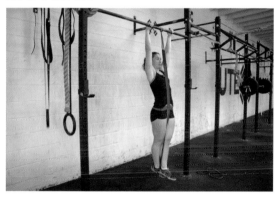 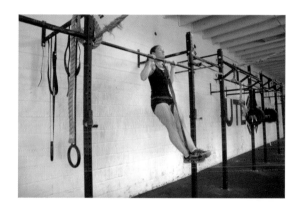

UNASSISTED PULL-UPS

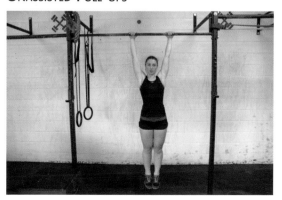 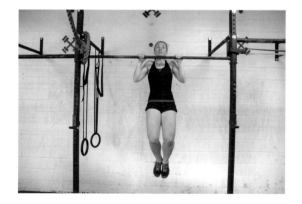

Broad Jumps

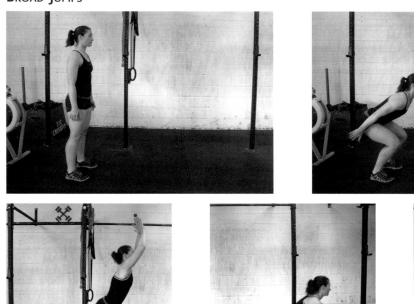

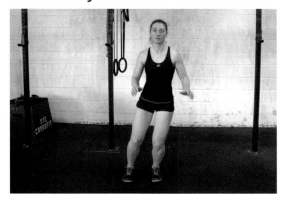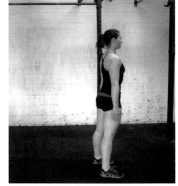

Side-to-Side Jumps

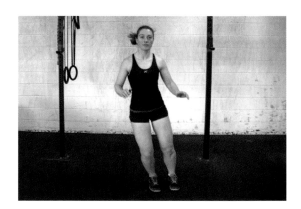

Box Jumps

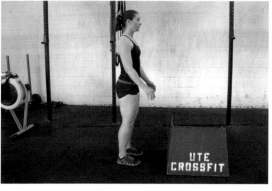 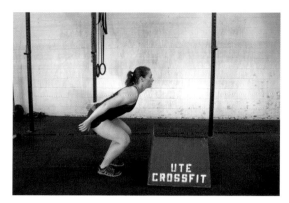

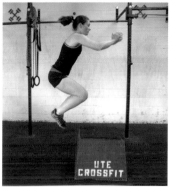 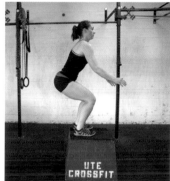 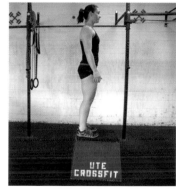

Dips

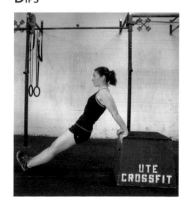 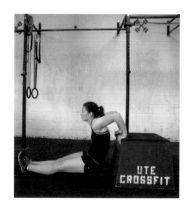 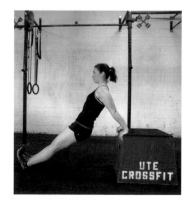

SIDE BENDS

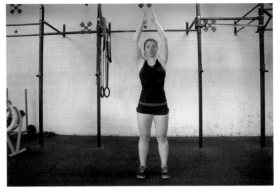 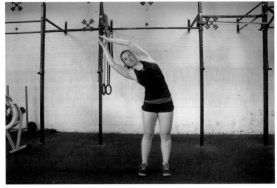

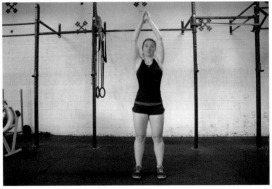 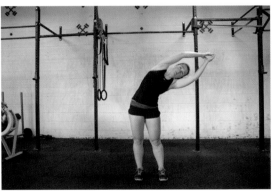

SIDE KICKS

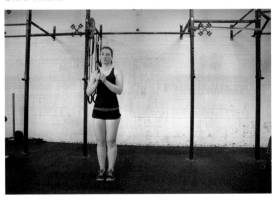 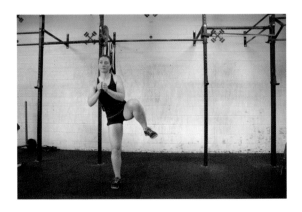

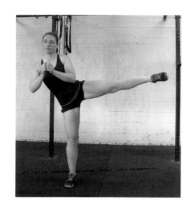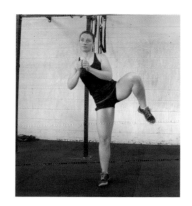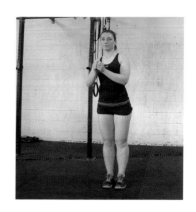

Pitfalls in Training

As you delve deeper into your process of getting off the couch and prepping to become race-ready, there are a few pitfalls to watch out for. The very first thing you must do is hide your scale, which can be your worst enemy in a training program, especially one focused on getting stronger. It is true that muscle weighs more than fat, so if you pack on muscle and melt away the fat you may in fact actually gain weight while losing inches. Instead of gauging your progress with pounds lost, gauge your progress by how your clothing fits. If the waistline of your favorite jeans feels a little bit looser towards the end of the month, then you are a bit leaner. If your pant legs seem to be a little bit tighter in the quads or thighs, it's a sign that your trail running is building muscle. Either way, the scale doesn't always show the same progress that the mirror does. Through your training, you just might fall in love with your body again.

The second pitfall that is seen time and time again is the dreaded plateau. A plateau occurs after your body has initially adapted to a workout routine. After a while, your body knows the drills, the trails and the training program, so you won't see the changes you saw in the initial weeks. This is a common occurrence in sports and training. The best way to combat a plateau is to vary your routine; it can be as simple as changing the time of day you train, or as complex as adding some increased intensity to your workouts. The reality is that plateaus do happen, so the best thing to do is watch for the warning signs, acknowledge them, and adjust accordingly.

Finally, the last major pitfall is overtraining. This goes back to the beginning of the chapter where I said you have to start slowly and build the foundation; overtraining is the result of doing the exact opposite. It is common among people looking to do it all at once, or former athletes who start their training program as if they just walked off the playing field. In both cases, overtraining does not make you stronger or faster, but can actually cause injury and fatigue. The most common cases of overtraining are those individuals who refuse to take days off for rest and recovery. This is the "more is better" model, when in reality more is just more, or worse. An effective one-hour high intensity workout in the gym can be as effective as someone else's three- to four-hour workout.

The first sign of overtraining is when you no longer are getting stronger or faster, as with a plateau, and even after varying your routines you still cannot improve. The second sign is sleeplessness, as overtraining has a way of taking away your ability to sleep. This robs the body of its time to recover and regenerate muscles. It's like a loop: you need to use energy in order to sleep, but you need sleep to have energy. Its the same with strength. When overtraining kicks in, you are no longer sleeping or getting stronger; you are just pushing forward. Often injuries arise in conjunction with overtraining due to the disruption of the loop. In the most extreme cases this sleeplessness can turn into nightmares—sometimes even night terrors—when you actually do sleep. Overtraining can become burn-out.

The good news is that overtraining is the simplest thing to combat! All you need to do to avoid overtraining is slow down and take a few days off. After a few days of your body relaxing, healing, and resting you will be back on the trails and in the gym prepping for your next race. Sometimes the best thing we can do for ourselves is to just relax a little, reflect on why we are doing it all, and come back to it with a renewed energy.

Finally, the biggest part of any training program is to simply have fun! Health and fitness are achieved at the highest levels when you love what you are doing. As you embark on your training journey, remember to smile when you succeed, laugh when you fall on your bum, and embrace the journey that is health and fitness. Once you do that, the changes that occur will not only be on the outside; you will also feel change from within.

"You are what you eat."

CHAPTER 6

CREATING A WINNING DIET

Two critical parts of any training program are nutrition and hydration, and both are often overlooked. The common fallacy, "I am working out so I can eat whatever I want" is heard over and over again. Many embark on a training program for just this purpose: train more to eat whatever you like. This, however, is not a sustainable way to build on the time and effort placed in your workouts each day.

Whole books are published daily about what you should or shouldn't eat. An entire book could be devoted just to nutrition for racing! This book offers a few key guidelines to help you physically achieve your best. The first thing is to throw out any preconceived ideas of what "diet" means. A favorite quote about diets comes from Garfield, "You know what a 'diet' is, don't you? It's 'DIE' with a 'T', that's what it is!" When the word is used, other words like "Atkins," "Paleo," "Zone," "Grapefruit," "Gluten-Free," "Popcorn," "California," or the names of hundreds of other designer, vogue or once-vogue fads pop up. Instead of thinking of a diet in terms of what you can or cannot eat, think of it instead as a nutritional compass, a barometer to help decide whether one food choice outweighs another in nutritional value.

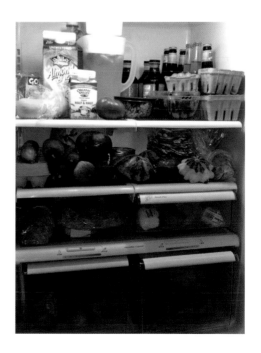

Instead of a strict set of rules, this book advocates a few simple guidelines for choosing what to eat. Simply, avoid processed food and instead replace them with whole foods, which

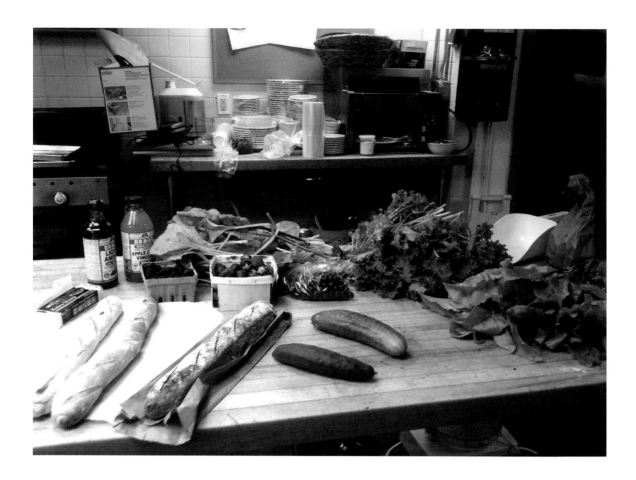

are nutrient-rich with little or no processing. The second step in creating a winning diet is to replace three large meals a day with five or six small meals. Research study after research study shows that those who consistently eat smaller meals more frequently are healthier and, especially in the case of athletes, maintain higher energy levels throughout the day.

Avoiding Processed Foods

Avoiding processed foods is easier than one might think. Even people on the most restricted budget can greatly decrease their processed food intake with a few simple detours in the grocery store. The secret of the grocery store is that everything you need is on the outside aisles. The perimeter of the store is where you find the fruits, vegetables, dairy, fresh bread, meats and fish. Basically, that is all you need to sustain yourself. Situated close to this perimeter are the bulk bins that contain the rice, beans, lentils, popcorn and other dried legumes. You can find all of this good, unprocessed food without stepping into about 80 percent of the store. Typically, the ever-growing "natural section" tends to be located on the outer aisles of the store as well. This almost systematically eliminates the need to enter most of the aisles, where almost all the processed stuff not needed in our diets is shelved. Next time you are in the grocery store, check it out.

In preparation for your first race, in addition to changing your food intake, you'll probably need to adjust your hydration. It is recommended that we all drink at least eight glasses of water a day; however, most American adults don't come close to that amount. Americans substitute water with things like coffee, tea, or sugared sports drinks. Just because a brand has "vitamin" in its name does not mean it is good for you! With the additional exercise in your daily routine your need for water will increase. A full gallon of water consumed each day will not only help you keep your diet on target by curbing cravings, but will also keep your system hydrated and functioning at a higher level. Two items can greatly help increase your water consumption: a gallon water jug and a water bottle.

In 2011, in preparation for a race, I knew I needed to ensure my water intake was sufficient for the full week leading up to the race. Each morning, I would fill the gallon jug with water. I would carry the jug around with me and by the end of the day would have finished it. This ensured I got the water I needed for the week. It is a practice I have continued, although I have swapped the muscle-head-gallon-jug look for a smaller water bottle. I do bring the jug to work with me and fill my water bottle from it throughout the day. At the end of the day I can gauge how I did on my hydration. It's a simple way to cut out the sugary drinks and instead replace them with healthy, clean water. Another way to boost hydration is to eat raw fruits and vegetables. Many plants contain a considerable amount of water, and it all helps.

Eat A Little A Lot

As children, most of us are taught to eat a big breakfast followed by a large lunch and another large meal for dinner. We were also often told not to snack in-between meals and instead to wait until it was "time to eat." Today, more and more researchers are debunking this old practice, especially for athletes. Instead of three large meals a day, athletes around the world are eating five or six smaller meals a day.

For many, this means a lot of planning during the day and a little bit of prep the night before so that you have what you need in the office on a workday. This practice also has many advantages. Eating six small meals a day ensures that your body will always have the nutrients it needs to function, decreases cravings for junk food, and increases your metabolic rate which, in return, helps you burn calories more efficiently. It can also help ward off that infamous mid-afternoon crash, because with six meals your blood sugar doesn't have significant lows.

To accomplish a successful six-meal day, include fiber, protein, and unsaturated fat in each meal. The meals should be about three hours apart and include at least two different food groups. The meals don't all need to be a huge ordeal; many think of the word "meal" and think of the dinners our parents served. The meals I am talking about are smaller. Breakfast might be an egg on wheat toast, a protein shake, or some Greek yogurt with fruit on top. The second meal of the day could be raw veggies with hummus or a cooked chicken breast with spinach. The key is that you are consuming the same number of calories over the course of the day as you did with three larger meals a day. The urge to grab that afternoon sweet or salty treat should be diminished.

As with a change in anything, the key is to start slowly. Your body needs the changes in your diet to happen progressively, just as with an exercise routine. If you have never eaten six many meals in a day, first try to decrease the portion size of your lunch and dinner. Focus on adding the mid-morning and mid-afternoon meals. These meals can start out as small snacks, easily accessible and easily prepared. As you become more comfortable with the changes in your diet, continue to decrease lunch and dinner to make the other meals equally prominent. If you're not in the habit of eating breakfast, you can start by adding in this meal to your day.

For those who have a current diet that consists of mostly processed and fast foods, the same starting rules apply. Ditch the white bread for more nutritious whole grain bread—one with lots of different grains in it. If you love your sweet snacks, many nutrition companies now offer great tasting powders that can help curb that craving and give you the protein you need to help build muscle mass, which in turn will get you through your first race.

Overall, the keys to a winning diet include eating often and in smaller portions, avoiding processed foods, and drinking enough water. These changes will help ensure that not only will you be more prepared for your first race, but soon you will also find that you are living a healthier life all around. Just remember that your eating habits and diet are always a work in progress. You might feel that you need to perfect your diet in order to finish a race. It's really a never-ending exploration of what your body wants and needs to help you perform at your best.

RECIPE

Sweet Treat – Chocolate Protein Cake

I have the world's biggest sweet tooth. I love cake and everything about it. Here is a healthier option to help curb that sweet crazing.

SERVINGS: 1

Ingredients:
1/2 scoop of protein powder
1 Tablespoon 100% cocoa powder
1/4 Tablespoon of baking soda
1/2 teaspoon of sugar
1 1/4 Tablespoon of applesauce
1 egg white

DIRECTIONS:
Mix dry ingredients together in a microwave safe mug or glass (tall mug is best). Mix in wet ingredients and stir until fully blended. Microwave for 1 minute on high. Remove form microwave and either eat it out of the mug or use a fork and gently loosen the cake from the mug and serve on a plate.

"Visualize this thing that you want, see it, feel it, believe in it. Make your mental blue print, and begin to build." – Robert Collier

CHAPTER 7

MENTAL PREPARATION

Yogi Berra once famously noted, of baseball and sports, that "90 percent is mental and the other half is physical." Many have laughed at this statement but Berra could have easily been talking about obstacle course racing. Few sports compare to OCR in the sheer amount of mental fortitude it takes to complete a race. However, with the right attitude, motivation, goal setting, mental imagery, stress management and concentration you can conquer your first race like a pro.

The first and most important aspect of obstacle course racing is having a positive attitude and being driven to use the race as an opportunity to learn something about yourself. As you prep for your first race it is important to keep the training and preparation in balance and perspective with the rest of your life. User whatever barriers in training and preparation may pop up as part of your training and keep a positive outlook on the process.

Motivation is the next most important thing. Why did you decide to do this race? Did you sign up with a group of friends or co-workers? What drives you to reach the finish line? What do you expect to get out of the race, other than a medal? It is important to take the time to self-assess after you sign up for a race. What do you really want out of it? You might not know

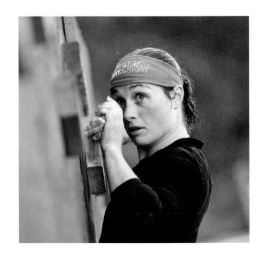

exactly what motivated you until after the event, but it's important to have an idea of why you want to be there; it makes the whole process more enjoyable.

Once you have established your motivation, then you can set a goal for yourself. Every first-time obstacle course racer should have the same goal: to complete the race. Finishing your first obstacle course race is an achievement—one that you will remember forever. People may have different definitions of what "finishing" means, but for your first race the most important thing should be not a ranking but rather the simple act of crossing the finish line. As you progress in the sport, the goal might evolve to finishing without a penalty, successful completion of all obstacles, or maybe one day to win a race or two. Be sure to write down your goals, put them in a place where you can constantly remind yourself what you are working for. This will help keep you more committed to the process of training and give you a specific objective to focus on.

In addition to your long-term goal of finishing the race, it is important to set short-term training goals along the way. These goals should be measurable and time-oriented. For example, if when starting your training program your personal best is ten sit-ups at a time, set your goal to completing twenty or thirty at a time without stopping by the end of week four. Or if, like me, you struggle with pull-ups, set a month-long goal of being able to do one or two pull-ups; to achieve this, add assisted pull-ups into each training session to gradually build the necessary muscle. These little short-term goals will help you step by step to reach your ultimate goal of finishing your first obstacle course race.

With your goals set and a clear vision of what you hope to succeed, the real preparation can start. Lifting the weights and physical training is actually the easy part, because a rarely talked about but important part of your training is mental imagery. As Robert Collier stated in the opening quote, in order to truly achieve your goals you need to see yourself doing them. Set aside the time to imagine yourself in a competition setting and mentally see yourself performing the skills and conquering the obstacles.

You can apply mental imagery to your daily training program. Before trying a particularly hard task, take 15 to 20 seconds and imagine successfully accomplishing that task. Close your eyes and create in your mind a detailed image of you succeeding, draw out the details, take note of the smells, sights and sounds around you. Let the feelings in as you draw your mental picture. Before you open your eyes, take in the whole picture, store it away, and then tackle the task. This is the first step in using mental imagery. Before each race, I use mental imagery to see myself accomplishing the obstacles. I picture how it looks and feels to climb over a wall. I set myself up mentally so I can physically accomplish the task the next morning. Even while racing, I imagine the successful completion of the obstacle before tackling it, especially in races where there are penalties for failed obstacles! If you have trouble visualizing what the obstacles might be like, check out old race videos and YouTube videos as a reference for what may lie ahead of you. Take those images and make them your own, seeing yourself in them, succeeding and pushing forward.

Once you start to use mental imagery in your training, it can even help you deal effectively with race day anxiety. Although such anxiety is to a large extent inevitable, it doesn't have to be a bad thing; it can in many cases be the catalyst that propels you past your perceived limits. One of the best exercises I've found for managing race day anxiety is a short mantra I have used with athletes for years: "calm, cool, collected." As you wait at the starting line, close your eyes for a few seconds, control your breathing, and silently repeat the phrase to yourself, as many times as you feel you need to. Take another deep breath, slowly open your eyes, and focus on leaving the starting line. With the use of mental imagery you can help keep your race day anxiety in check and perform at your best.

The next step in your mental journey is to acknowledge that you will face a range of emotions. You need to realize and accept that you will feel excitement, anger and disappointment, sometimes all within the span of a few minutes during an obstacle course race. Instead of letting each emotion take over, acknowledge it, accept it, and then move on. Refocus your energies on the task at hand. While any OCR is sure to be an eventful day, the most action and the greatest challenges you will face are going on in your head, not out on the course.

In the 2011 World's Toughest Mudder, I didn't think about crossing the finish line when I started the 24-hour race. I took it one lap at a time. When that became too overwhelming, I took it one obstacle at a time; in the last couple of hours of racing I was taking the race one step at a time. There is no end-goal we can't accomplish if we break it up, slow it down and put one foot in front of the other. When I even for a minute thought about the race as a whole it seemed unachievable, but taking it in pieces I went further than I ever had before. Since then I have used this technique in multiple ultra-marathons, obstacle course races, and in daily life when a to-do list seems too daunting.

Finally, the last obstacle is to mentally conquer is your own fear. Many runners stay away from obstacle course races fearing injury and the obstacles themselves. You will most likely walk away from a race with a few scrapes and some bruises but nothing more. Obstacle course racing is as safe as many trail races, I personally have tumbled more often off trails during a trail race than an obstacle course race. Do not let the fear of the obstacles overtake you.

Many people express fear of obstacles containing electricity. The race organizer that is best known for electricity in their obstacles is Tough Mudder. The voltage is high and the internet is filled with videos of the obstacle taking participants down. However, as you will read in Chapter 8, if you move quickly through the obstacle it won't hurt you. Instead of fearing obstacles going into race day, use the visualization exercises to see yourself successfully completing the obstacle. The more you visualize success, the more you will actualize it on race day.

Ultimately, the key to mentally preparing yourself for your first obstacle course race is to throw out expectations, keep yourself committed to your goals (both big and small), and practice some self-talk and concentration. With that in place, you will be head and shoulders ahead of your competition at the starting line, ready to conquer anything that lies ahead.

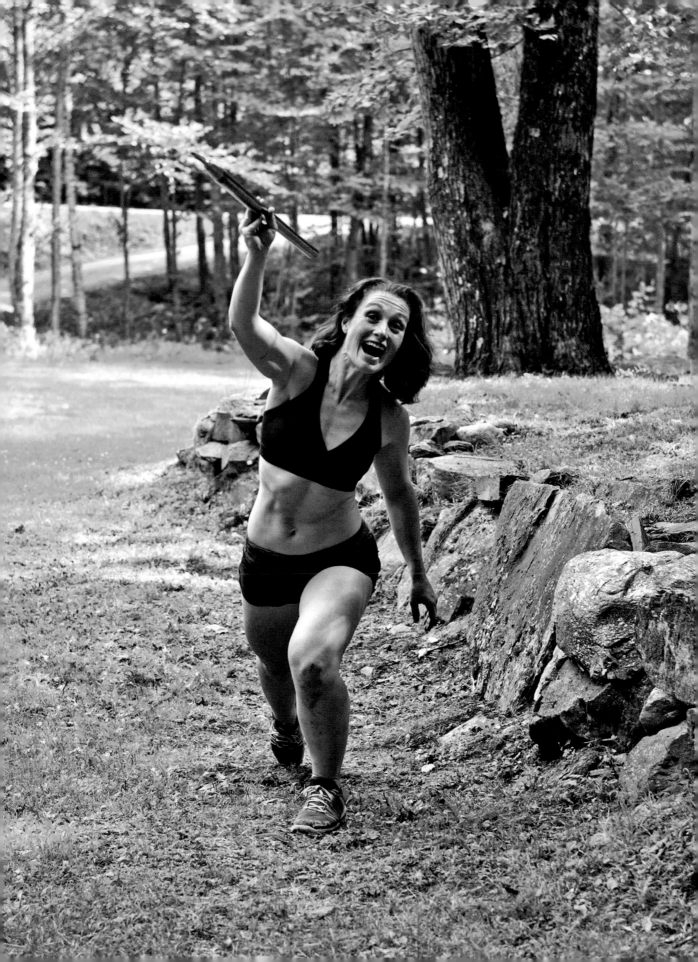

SECTION 3

MASTERING THE COURSE

The obstacles have always been my friend in racing. When I started in the OCR circuit, it was the obstacles that drew my non-runner self into each race; they broke up the running portions, which I found more challenging, so even the toughest obstacle still seemed like a relief to me! With that said, it took years of racing before I was able to run a clean race in the Spartan Race series and a long time before I was able to complete all the obstacles unassisted.

For years, my arch nemesis was the spear throw obstacle. I went over two seasons without being able to successfully complete this obstacle. It got to the point where I built a wall, spear, and target in my back yard to practice. I was determined to finally succeed at that obstacle. In the summer of 2012 I spent every morning drinking coffee and throwing spears in my backyard. Luckily, I lived in the wood, with no neighbors in sight to wonder what the crazy woman next door was doing. Ultimately, the hard work and practice time paid off later that summer when finally, after over two years of racing, I succeeded at my first spear throw in a race; I wanted to jump up and down when I hit the target, but the race had to go on so I kept running. The elation I felt that day after so many missed attempts was a highlight of the summer. It isn't the memory of the podium placement I earned that day that sticks with me, but the fact that I finally nailed the spear throw.

The more races I go to, the more I realize that the successful completion of obstacles has more to do with believing you can complete them than with physical skill. In winter 2013, while racing in the Fuego y Agua Survival Run, a 75K jungle obstacle race, I reached an obstacle in which I needed to climb 25 feet up a tree to retrieve one of only a few available wristbands before I could continue to the next obstacle. There was no safety net below, just a concrete slab. The margin of error was slim to none. I stood there not sure of my skills but knowing it had to be done. I had a film crew in my face as I nervously looked up at what needed to happen but calmly told the camera, "This is one of those times in life you need to turn off the brain and just do it." After an initial quick attempt with my mind not in the right place, I failed. I regrouped, selected another tree and knew I had one chance to make it happen (those wristbands were going fast…). In many ways I left my own self for a few minutes, shut down the fear and doubt and just moved. I scaled higher in that tree than I had ever been before, shaking as I grasped the wristband, and quickly climbed down the coconut tree; I had accomplished it. I had gone beyond what I had ever thought myself capable of, and succeeded.

Whether it is a 5-foot wall, spear throw or scaling a coconut tree, you will surprise yourself with what you can accomplish and how far beyond what you thought possible your body can go. You too can master the course during your first race!

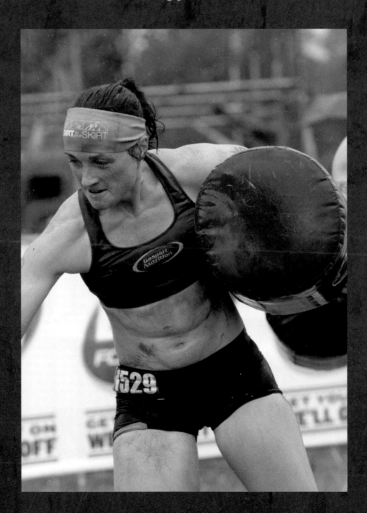

CHAPTER 8

THE OBSTACLES

In this chapter, we introduce and explain how to get through some of the most-asked-about race obstacles. Although obstacles vary from event to event, there is a standard set of obstacles that seems to have taken hold of the sport. Each of the following obstacles is explained in such a way that you can practice the necessary skills in a gym environment leading up to a race. With a little bit of extra practice, you can truly excel at your first race.

Eight-Foot and Ten-Foot Walls

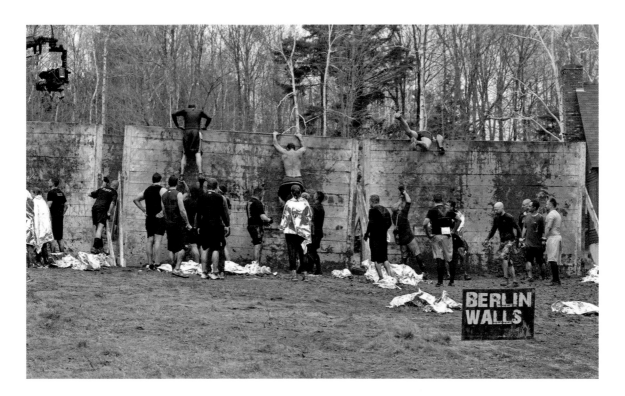

Eight-foot walls tend to be one of the biggest hurdles for many racers, and it is common for racers to struggle to find creative ways over the walls. If you are racing with a few people I recommend that you help each other over these walls (i.e., boost one or more people up the wall, who will help to pull the rest of you over). However, if you are racing alone there are two ways to get over the wall, depending whether there is a helper step (mostly only for women) or not. Most walls under eight-feet do not have a helper step so try the following how-tos.

Wall without Helper Step

STEP 1
As you approach the obstacle, eye the spot on the wall where you will want to plant your foot. You will want to aim for a target about waist high.

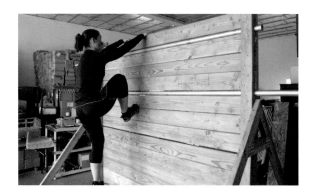

STEP 2
Run towards the wall with a little speed. Maintain even strides and a consistent pace as you approach the wall.

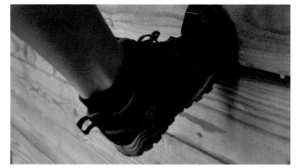

STEP 3
Jump up and forward off your left leg (or non-dominant side), as if you are doing a long skip. You should take off on your jump about a meter or so away from the wall, but this distance can vary depending on your height and size.

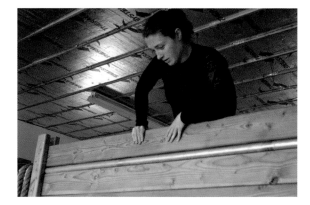

STEP 4

Plant the ball of your dominant foot on the wall where you eyed it. At the same time, thrust your other leg up hard.

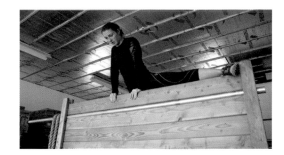

STEP 5

Extend your arms and shoulders up to get momentum while pushing up. Reach and grab the top of the wall tightly; if you can, try to plant your forearm on top of the wall.

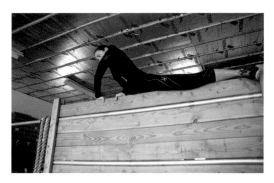

STEP 6

Pull yourself up (using your forearm to brace yourself, if possible) and press up with the other hand so that your hips are now parallel with the top of the wall.

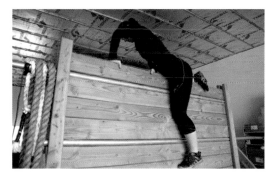

STEP 7

Brace your weight forward and balance on the wall, lift one leg up and over the wall. You should end up in a straddled position with one leg on either side of the wall.

STEP 8

Shift your hands so that you are now facing the side you just came from. Then swing your other leg over and lower your body to the ground.

Walls with Helper Step

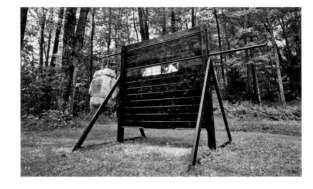

STEP 1
Eye the spot on the wall where the helper step is located. It should be a small block of wood sticking out a few inches from the wall.

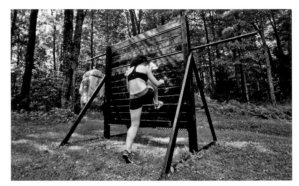

STEP 2
Run towards the wall with a little speed. You will want to have even strides and a consistent pace as you approach the wall.

STEP 3
Jump up and forward off your left leg (or non-dominant side), like you are doing long skip. You should take off on your jump about a meter or so away from the wall, but this can vary due to height and size.

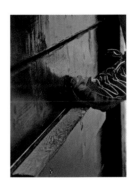

STEP 4
"Toe" into the block on the wall as you would if you were rock climbing. Extend your arms and shoulders up to get momentum while "toeing" in. Reach and grab the top of the wall tightly.

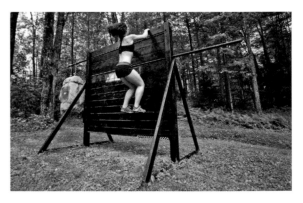

STEP 5

Match your back toe onto the helper block and with both feet jump up, while at the same time pressing down with your hands to raise your waist to become level with the top of the wall.

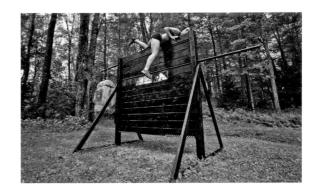

STEP 6

Shift your body weight forward and balance on the wall; lift one leg up and over the wall. You should complete this step in a straddled position with one leg on either side of the wall.

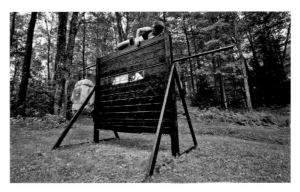

STEP 7

Shift your hands so that you are now facing the side you just came from. Then swing your other leg over and lower your body to the ground.

Gym Exercise:

If you do not have a wall readily accessible, there are a few gym exercises that can help build the strength needed to master this obstacle. The two best exercises to help in your training are strict pull-ups (the non-kipping kind) and muscle-ups. If you cannot perform a full pull-up, start by modifying the exercise with an exercise band, or place a box under the bar and do jumping pull-ups. Jumping pull-ups are great for working explosiveness and building strength.

Rope Climb

The rope climb is a traditional obstacle in obstacle course racing. Most races have either a knotted or unknotted climb in it. The unknotted climbing technique can be used for both knotted and unknotted ropes; however, when you are presented with a knotted rope you'll want to use those knots to your advantage.

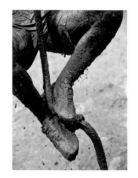

Rope Climb with Knots

STEP 1

Grab the rope with both hands above the highest knot possible.

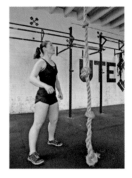

STEP 2

Pull down on the rope while jumping a bit, so you are lifted into the air (or out of the water pit, in many races).

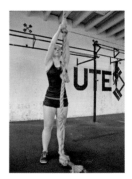

STEP 3

Reach your arms up as high as you can and grip the rope tightly.

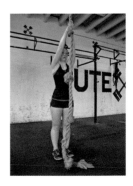

STEP 4

Using your core (abdominal muscles), bring your knees up to your chest, finding the highest comfortable knot.

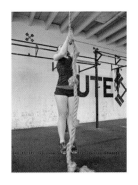

STEP 5

Pinch the arches of your shoes around the knot, cupping the knot and giving you a platform to stand on.

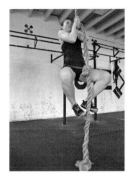

STEP 6

Stand up with your legs, and reach as high as possible with your arms.

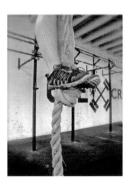

STEP 7

Repeat steps 4 through 7 until you reach the top of the rope. In many races you will reach for a bell in order to prove you truly reached the top of the rope.

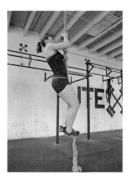

STEP 8

Use the knots to climb back down, lowering your body knot by knot. If you are afraid of heights, you can literally sit on the knots as you lower yourself down.

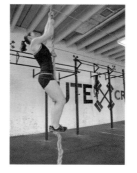
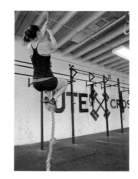

Rope Climb without Knots

STEP 1

Grab the rope with both hands above your head.

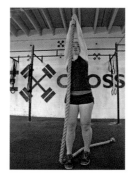

STEP 2

Pull down on the rope while jumping a bit, so you are lifted into the air (or out of the water pit in many races).

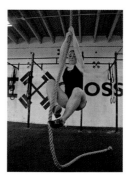

STEP 3

Wrap the rope around one leg, and use your feet to pinch the rope, thus anchoring yourself.

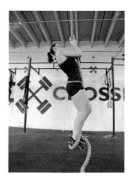

STEP 4

Reach your arms up as high as you can and grip the rope tightly.

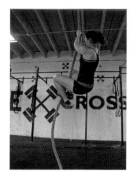

STEP 5

Release the rope from your feet. Using your core (abdominal muscles), bring your knees up to your chest. Repeat step 3 with your feet.

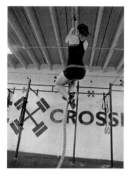

STEP 6

Stand up with your legs, and re-reach as high as possible with your arms.

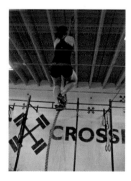

STEP 7

Repeat this "inch-worm" process until you have reached the top of the rope. In many races you will reach for a bell in order to prove you truly reached the top of the rope.

STEP 8

Loosen the grip of your feet on the rope when coming down. Support your weight evenly between your feet and hands. Slide your feet down, lower yourself slowly, placing hand under hand on the way down.

Gym Exercise:

If your gym has climbing ropes great—it is always best to practice on the actual obstacle you will encounter in a race. If your training space does not have a climbing rope, you can work on a variety of shoulder press exercises to help build your upper body strength. Again, pull-ups will also help to increase your grip and upper body strength. Good range of motion and flexibility will help you maneuver up the knots as well.

Barbed Wire

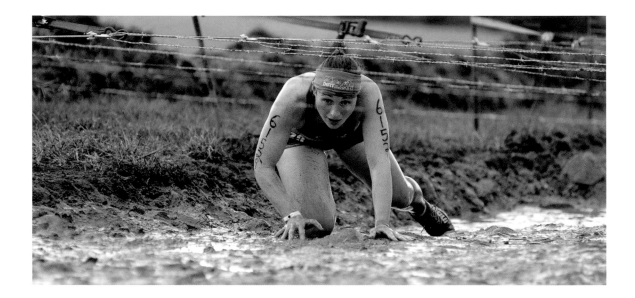

Barbed Wire Crawl & Roll

Barbed wire is a staple of obstacle course racing, whether it is the real thing or simply a cord strung across a road or mud pit. It really isn't an obstacle course race without at least one muddy pit you need to cross. The two most popular choices for navigating these muddy pits are the log roll or the traditional low or army crawl. Either rolling or crawling may be faster, depending the type of the terrain and whether any extra obstacles[22] are placed in the way.

---

22 Extra obstacles could be anything from bales of hay or boulders designed to impede a straight roll, a mud pit placed in the middle of a longer barbed wire section or, in one race in Texas, actual cacti dispersed in the barbed wire.

Roll

This is arguably the easier way through this obstacle. You simply lie down on your stomach, with your body perpendicular to the direction of the trail, and proceed to roll your body through the obstacle, making sure to keep your arms close to your chest as you roll. Find a fixed spot to focus your gaze on to minimize dizziness. If you need to stop due to dizziness pull off to the side of the obstacle wire and rest. Be careful when exiting to not get caught in the last of the barbed wire.

This is the best technique for extra low barbed wire or taller people. Shorter racers may find the next option to be a better technique.

Roll

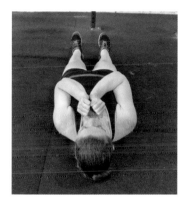 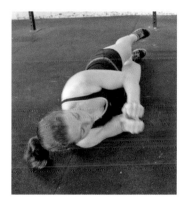 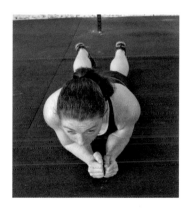

Low Crawl

The most important factor when employing the crawl is to keep a tight core and keep your back and butt down, similar to a push-up or plank position.

LOW CRAWL
STEP 1
Start by lying down on your stomach or in a push-up position as you enter the barbed wire area.

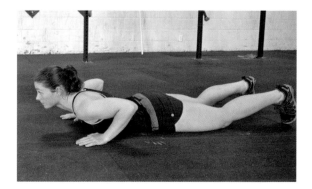

STEP 2

Start by bringing up your right leg (for viewing purposes, we're showing all moves from the left side) along the right side of your torso. You should almost feel like you can touch your right elbow with your knee.

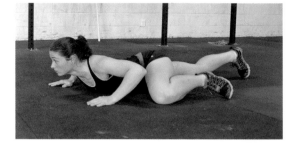

STEP 3

Reach your left arm (opposite side) forward above your head, with your elbow bent at 90 degrees, and resting your weight on your elbow and forearm. If the terrain is really rocky, you can use your hands, but remember to stay low.

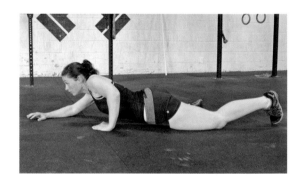

STEP 4

Transfer your weight to the bent right leg and forward left elbow/hand and push your torso ahead until your body comes in contact with your left arm and your legs are both even and extended.

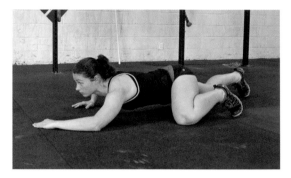

STEP 5

Repeat with the other leg and arm. As you crawl forward with opposing legs/arms, keep your hips and shoulders at the same height. Try not to lift your hips and (not to mention your head!) as you shift your weight forward, as this could put you in contact with the barded wire.

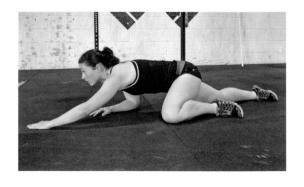

Bear Crawl

If you are small enough or the wire is high enough you can employ the bear crawl, a higher variation of the low crawl.

BEAR CRAWL

STEP 1

Drop to your hands and knees on the ground. Your knees should be directly under your hips and your hands directly under your shoulders. Make sure to engage your core muscles and straighten your back.

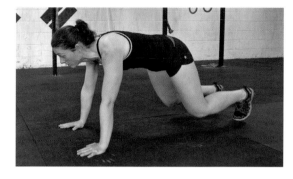

STEP 2

Reach forward with the right arm and right knee. Once the right hand and knee are planted on the ground, shift your body weight forward and prepare to reach out your left arm and left knee.

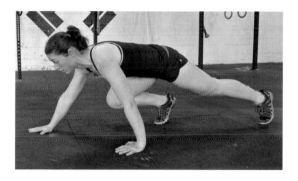

STEP 3

Continue to keep your core muscles engaged as you reach your left arm and left knee forward, shifting your weight over from the right side of your body.

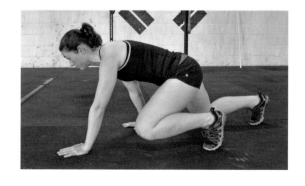

STEP 4

Alternate the movement from side to side. Continue to alternate this crawling sequence utilizing the same side arm and leg until you are out of the barbed wire area.

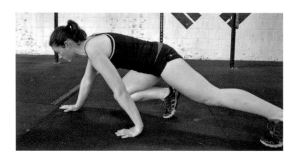 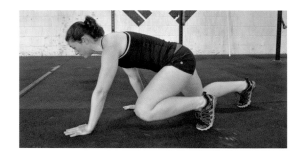

Gym Exercises:

All of the movements above can be practiced in the gym or at your local field. It is highly recommended that you practice the two types of crawls and get comfortable with the roll. Incorporate crawling into weekly workouts and you will see results at your race. The other two key body movements to developing your crawling strength are push-ups and a variation of the push-up called a dive bomber push-up (which involves a duck and dive movement like prone cobra in yoga).

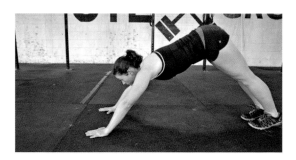 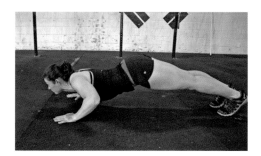

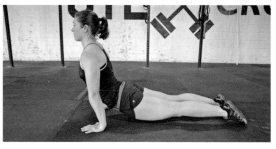

Tyrolean Traverse

The Tyrolean Traverse is a less common obstacle and thus becomes harder to conquer when it does appear in certain races. It is essentially a single rope slung between two points,

which you can cross either by hanging under the rope or resting your body on top of it. Either method will get you across it and both should be practiced. Hanging under the rope will require more physical exertion than crossing on top of it; however, either can be faster for you, depending on your body strength.

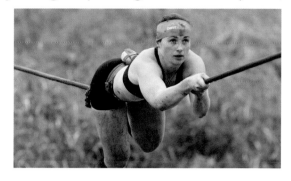

Monkey Crawl Method (body below the rope)

MONKEY CRAWL

STEP 1

Grasp the rope with both hands and swing your legs up and over top of the rope. Your head should face the direction you are going.

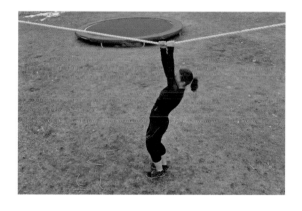

STEP 2

Pull your body weight along the rope with your hands and push with your feet, alternating them as you move forward.

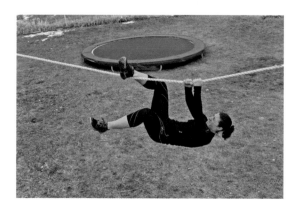

STEP 3

At the end of the rope (or at the bell you are required to ring), maintain your grip but release your legs, dropping to the ground or water below.

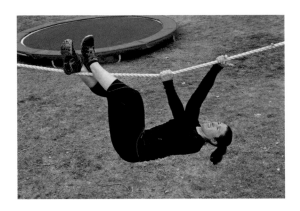 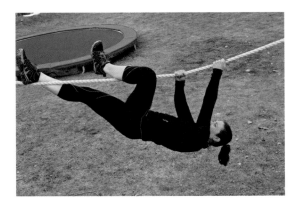

Commando Crawl Method (body above the rope)

STEP 1

Lie on the top of the rope with one foot hooked around it. Use the other foot as a counterbalance.

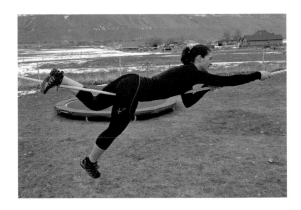

STEP 2

Keep the hooked foot bent and close to your butt.

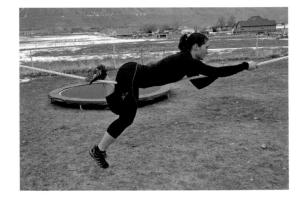

STEP 3

Pull your body along the rope using the anchor leg for balance throughtout. If you are wearing a hydration belt, make sure to slide the buckle to the side before attempting this obstacle.

STEP 4

Pull yourself forward with an overhand or underhand grip using your hands and arm strength.

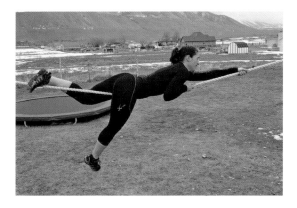

STEP 5

At the end of the rope (or at the obstacle bell), flip your body over, hang from your hands and drop onto the ground or into water below.

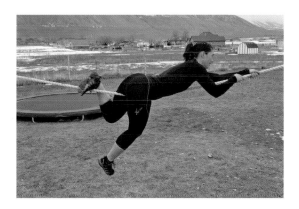

Gym Exercise:

This obstacle is best achieved with upper body strength to pull you along the rope. Any exercises in which you are pulling weights, or dragging sleds or other objects, will help build these muscles. One exercise you can do involves a tire and a rope: find a truck or small tractor tire, tie a rope around it and give it about 20 feet of slack that you can pull. Walk away from the tire until the rope is taut, then pull the tire to you, using your arms. This exercise will simultaneously strengthen your lower body as you brace yourself and work your upper body.

Spear Throw

The spear throw is synonymous with the Spartan Race, although other events have recently added obstacles like this one. It is one of the few obstacles that can be improved upon only with specific practice; there is no substitute. And a missed spear throw in a Spartan Race could cost you a 30 burpee penalty.

STEP 1

When you reach the spear throw obstacle, you will find a stack of spears on the ground and a target approximately 10 to 20 feet away. Your first challenge is to find the cleanest spear, or the one with the least amount of mud on it. This will ensure you have the best grip possible, reducing the chances of it slipping out of your hand when you're throwing.

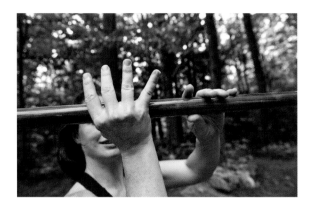

STEP 2

Once you have selected your spear, you will want to find the center balance point on the handle. Hold the spear loosely in your hand and find where it seems to balance parallel to the ground. This is where you want to grip the handle. Imagine playing (giant) darts.

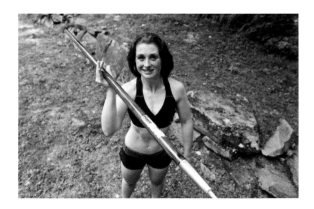

STEP 3

Grip the spear loosely in your dominant hand. Hold the spear at ear height, level it, and aim at your target. Take a deep breath, relax and visualize the spear hitting the target.

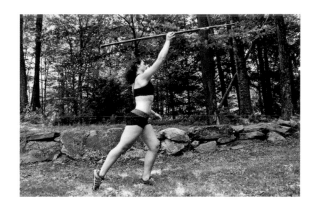

STEP 4

As you initiate the throw, step your non-dominant foot (i.e., your left foot if you are right-handed) forward. Use the power in your back leg to give you momentum as you release the spear. Some prefer a running start, believing it increases power. This technique requires much more skill in timing and is actually harder and requires much more practice. I advocate the standing start for beginners.

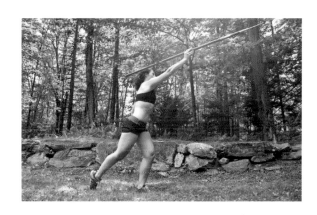

STEP 5

The trick to the spear throw is making minimal wrist movement with the release of the spear. This will allow the spear to fly straight in the air. The throw is much like that of a dart. The spear will go wherever you point your throwing arm.

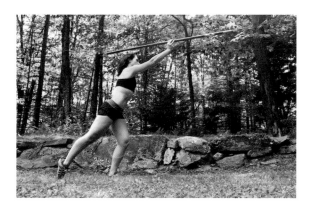

STEP 6

Watch it fly through the air and hit the target, then move on to the next obstacle! Do NOT run out into the range to retrieve your spear, and do NOT throw while spears are being collected.

Gym Exercise:

Again, there isn't any particular exercise that will help you conquer this obstacle; you need to practice doing the real thing. The best you can do in the gym is strengthen your grip and forearm muscles to help you throw straight when you are fatigued.

Obstacles Discussed:

The obstacles covered above are the ones that most people hardest with, but they represent only a small sampling of what you may see in a given race. Most races will also include some of the following obstacles for you to navigate through. Many are simple and require little practice, while others test your mental strength and fortitude more than your physical strength.

Cargo Nets

Whether they are placed vertically or horizontally, in a pyramid shape or straight up in the air, cargo nets are common. The best way to approach a cargo net is to climb either near a side, if you are not afraid of heights, or near a center support. Cargo nets sag and if you are able to stay near the edge the rope will be tighter and it will be easier to get your footing.

Carrying Objects

It is common for race organizers to include one of these strength-based obstacles; whether you are carrying a sandbag, bucket full of sand, rock, log or tires, it is a certainty that at some point you will be carrying something. The important thing to remember in these obstacles is to squat down when picking up the object and use the power in your legs to pick it up. This will help save your back from any strain.

Cliff Jump/High Jump/Walk the Plank/Leap of Faith

The name of the obstacle depends on the race, but in the end it's all the same thing: you reach a point in the race where you find yourself on a platform, and you must jump 10 to

20 feet below into a pool of water. This is an obstacle where it is best not to think, stop or worry. The best technique here is to just step up, look straight ahead (not down) and jump. The longer you think about it, the easier it is to psych yourself out. If you cannot swim or have a fear of heights, races either offer lifejackets or a bypass option.

Electric Shock

The electrified obstacles are most common in the Tough Mudder series but other events are adopting them as well. These obstacles are more mental than anything else. The "Electric Shock Therapy" obstacle is a section you run though. Electrified wires hang down, running high voltage in short spurts. It all sounds scary but in reality if you just run through quickly with your hands in front of you (try to avoid swinging your arms), you may feel a few pops but will get through it with ease. Do not stop or slow down while running the obstacle. If you have heart problems, you will want to skip this one.

Everest Quarter Pipe

The Everest Quarter-Pipe originated with Tough Mudder; other races have since adapted their own versions. The obstacle looks like a skateboard quarter-pipe. Depending on the size of the pipe, you may need assistance completing it. It is best to gain speed running into it, then use one foot to jump up hard, and reach for and grab the top of the ramp. In most Tough Mudders, people who reach the top successfully wait and help fellow competitors to complete this obstacle.

Fire Leap

The fire leap may be one of the easiest obstacles but often causes many racers a lot of anxiety. The key is that the flames are not what burn you; the coals underneath are really what you need to watch out for. The easiest way over this obstacle is to continue to run and leap, like a ballet dancer. Whether it looks graceful or no, it will get you over the fire. I have even seen people basically walk over the fire. It is such a short time that it will not hurt you (and you are often soaking wet at this point, so even less at risk).

Gladiators

Gladiators with pugil sticks are an iconic part of the Spartan Race series, though they sometimes appear at other races too. This is typically the very last obstacle, immediately before the finish line. These gladiators are normally muscular men, but sometimes women, who look to block your path or hit you with the foam ends of the pugil sticks as you approach. If you don't want to be hit hard, then don't run in looking for a fight. The gladiators tend to be more aggressive the more aggressively you act towards them. If you run in just looking to finish a fun race they will be much kinder to you!

Ice Water Baths

Depending on the location of the race these can either be a shock to the system or a nice relief from the heat. Either way, the best way to tackle a container full of ice water is to jump right in. It is much easier on the body than inching your way in. The faster you move through the water, the sooner this obstacle is over! Once you are out of the water, particularly if it is a cold day, shake out your arms and legs as you resume your run. It will help the blood flow back into your cold extremities.

Incline Walls

Incline walls normally have a rope hanging down to aid you in climbing over them, or they may have blocks to give you foot-and hand holds. If there is a rope, look for one with knots if possible; if there are no knots, wrap your arm around the rope when using it to climb. As you climb lean back and sit back a little bit/squat slightly as you go. When you get towards the top you will want to swing one leg over the wall. Once you've hooked your leg, you can pull the rest of your body up and over the wall.

Monkey Bars

Whether they are angled, straight, uneven or some other design, monkey bars are the obstacle that brings back childhood playground memories. Each race has its own take on monkey bars. The key is to keep your arms bent a little when swinging from bar to bar. Many times the bars are oddly spaced so it's best to match hand to hand instead of attempting large sweeping swings across.

Mud Pits

Mud pits vary greatly from race to race; some you can jump over, in some you scale a small mound of dirt and descend into muddy water, and others are just holes dug in the ground. The most important thing when entering a muddy pit is to go in feet first and use your arms for balance. The pit may be one depth throughout, or depth may vary from spot to spot; since you will not be able to see your feet, take one high step in front of the other until you are out of the pit. Be careful with the bottom of the pit; there are often roots to get caught on, and the muddy floor has been known to suck racers' shoes off their feet if they aren't careful!

Over-Under-Throughs

These are a series of obstacles that require you to go over a small wall, normally about four feet high, then under a wall with a foot and a half opening, then through a third wall with square holes. These normally come in sets of one or two. When going under the second wall, many find it easier to roll rather than crawl. When going through the third wall, grab onto the top braces, and step through or slip your legs through the hole first.

Pipe Crawls/Trenches

This is another obstacle that is more psychological than physical. You will want to either low crawl or bear crawl through these as you would in a barbed wire obstacle. Often the pipes or trenches zigzag, so you can't see any light while climbing through them. The best thing is to do is keep moving forward, not stopping until the end. Eventually you will reach light and you will complete it!

Slides

Slides are one of the easiest and most fun obstacles in any race. They require no effort and you get to laugh as you slide down adult versions of slip-n-slides. It is best to do this obstacle sitting up with your feet first. Then you just smile for the camera!

Tractor Tire Flip

The tire flip is making its way into more and more races. If you have not tried this before, when you come to the obstacle ask the volunteer which tire, if there are multiple to choose from, is the lightest. Use the power in your legs to lift the tire and flip it. Don't despair if you cannot do it on your own; racers often work in pairs.

Tractor Pull

The Tractor Pull is another Spartan Race staple. A chain is attached to a heavy cinder block, which you are instructed to drag around part of the marked course anywhere from a couple hundred feet to almost a quarter or half mile. The key is to tie a knot in the end of the chain to help keep your hand from slipping. Also, lock one hand near your hip to help move the weight forward.

Wall Traverse

The wall traverse is becoming increasingly popular, whether the walls have rock-climbing holds or simply blocks of wood you use to traverse yourself across the wall. The key to success here is to strengthen your grip, and keep your hips as close to the wall as possible. A great way to practice this skill is to find a local climbing gym and practice bouldering.

Water/Swims

Most water or swimming obstacles you will encounter in races are not very deep (most are waist to chest high), and race organizers often offer a bypass or provide lifejackets for those who are nervous about swimming. The swims are fun, but like the ice bath obstacles, after you get out of them make sure you shake out your arms and legs to get blood pumping back through them before moving onto the next obstacle.

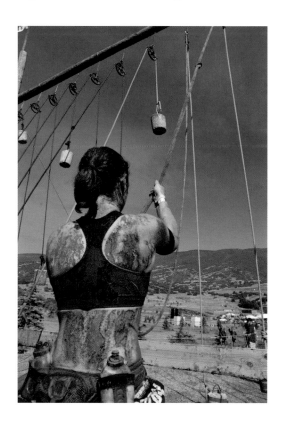

CHAPTER 9

THE GREAT BURPEE DEBATE

Love them or hate them, the burpee is one of the most infamous exercises in all of obstacle racing. At just the mention of the word many shudder, while others feel elated by the challenge. Whichever side of the debate you are on, this is one exercise you should get comfortable with. The fitness world has many variations and definitions of what the "correct" burpee is; some include a push-up while others do not, and some include a jump and in others you just stand up. No matter how you define the burpee, it's been around a long time. Recently, with the rise of obstacle course racing, CrossFit and other functional lifting programs, it seems to have come back into vogue again.

So what is a burpee? Simply put, a burpee is a body weight exercise that consists of stringing several movements together to form a full body exercise that uses strength and explosive power. The Oxford Dictionary defines a burpee as "a physical exercise consisting of a squat thrust made from and ending in a standing position." The burpee draws it origins from an American psychologist named Royal H. Burpee. In the 1930s he developed the "Burpee Test" to gauge subjects' fitness levels. The Burpee Test consisted of a series of burpees performed in rapid succession to measure agility and coordination. It became popular during World War II when the United States Armed Services adopted it as a way to assess the fitness level of recruits. Today, it's seen on obstacle course races, in CrossFit gyms and all over the world as a great full-body workout with no added equipment.

There are many variations of the burpee ranging in intensity, from the basic version for beginners to some very creative and difficult ones for professional athletes. They include the knee push-up, jump up, tuck-jump, jump-over, box-jump, one-armed, dumbbell, parkour, Hindu push-up, muscle-up, double, one leg, side variation, as well as wall or incline or air burpee. All of these types build on the same basic foundational movements, described on page 90.

Original Four-Count Burpee:
1. Start standing up.
2. Place your hands on the ground in squat position.
3. Kick your legs out behind you into plank position.
4. Return to squat position, hands on the ground.
5. Return to standing position.

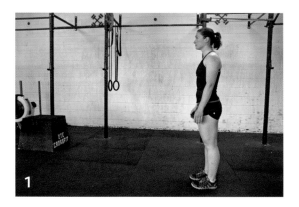

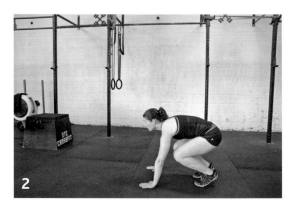

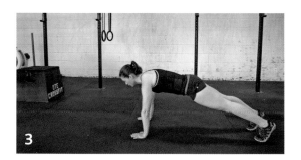

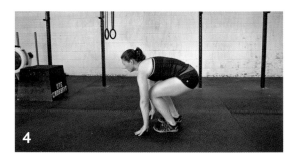

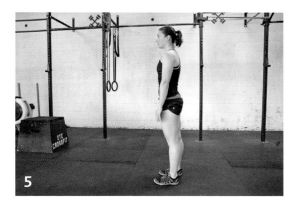

Eight-Count Burpee:

1. Start standing up.
2. Place your hands on the ground in squat position.
3. Kick your legs out behind you into plank position.
4. Lower your body for a push-up.
5. Raise your body up from the push-up, returning to plank position.
6. Return to squat position, hands on the ground.
7. Stand up.

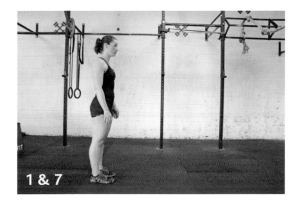

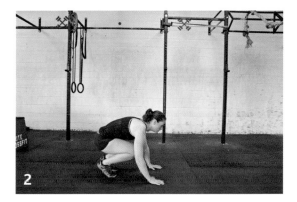

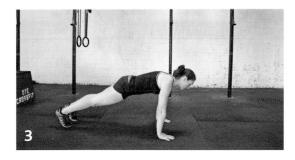

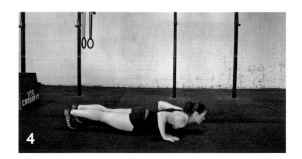

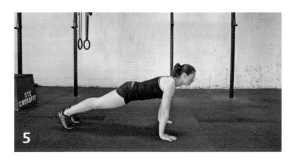

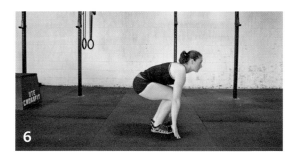

8. Jump up in the air and clap hands together overhead.
9. Return to standing position.

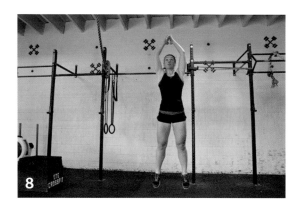

Long Jump Burpee

1. Start standing up.
2. Place your hands on the ground in squat position.
3. Kick your legs out behind you into plank position.
4. Lower your body for a push-up.
5. Raise your body up from the push-up, returning to plank position.
6. Return to squat position, hands on the ground.
7. Stand up.
8. Complete a broad jump forward for distance.
9. Return to standing position.

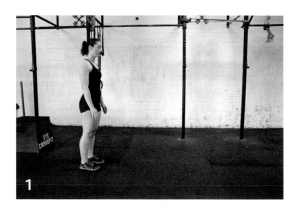 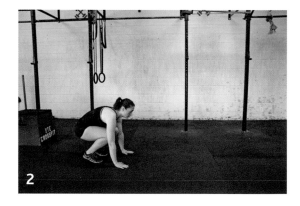

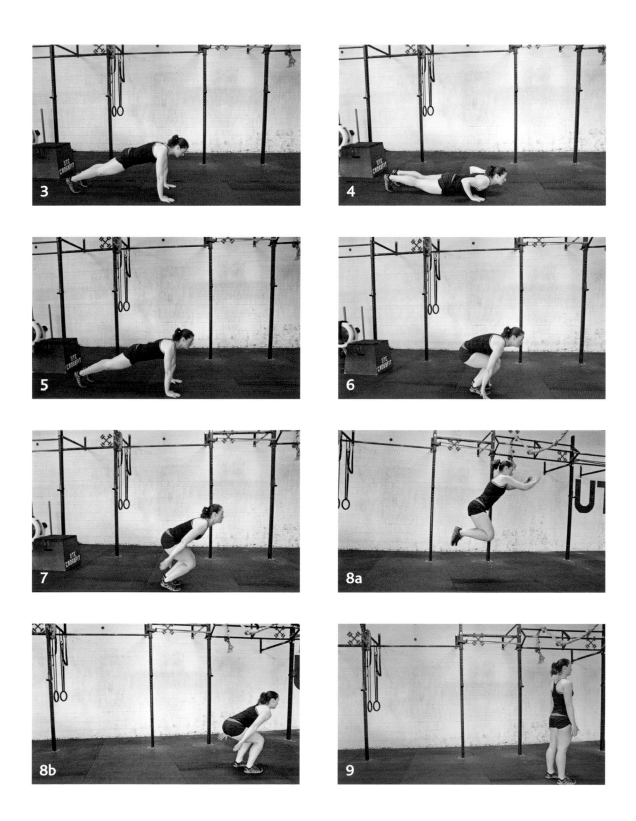

Pull-Up Burpee (follow the illustrations for the eight-count purpee through step 7)
1. Start standing up.
2. Place your hands on the ground in squat position.
3. Kick your legs out behind you into plank position.
4. Lower your body for a push-up.
5. Raise your body up from the push-up, returning to plank position.
6. Return to squat position, hands on the ground.
7. Stand up.
8. Jump up to grip an overhead bar and complete a pull-up. (see lower right photo on p. 47 for technique).
9. Return to standing position.

The two most popular versions today are the Eight-Count Burpee or the Military Eight-Count Bodybuilder, which includes the push-up and jump or jump and clap. Each variation can be challenging and gives everyone a chance to experience the pleasure and pain of the burpee.

Obstacle course racing has seen a huge evolution in burpees in the last couple of years. Some races, like the Spartan Race, use the burpee as a penalty for failed obstacles, while other races like the Civilian Military Combine use it as part of the race itself. Most races use the four-count burpee as their official burpee. In 2012, the Spartan Race modified its rules to make the official burpee the eight-count version, with or without the clap.

There is no doubt that as races are becoming increasingly more creative, more burpee variations will follow. This was evident in 2012 at the Spartan Race held in Fenway Park, where the exercise was not only the penalty for a failed obstacle, but was also incorporated into obstacles by design; even a 30-burpee station was added. The race organizers only get more and more creative each year, so the best thing you can do is prepare yourself.

In the end, it doesn't matter which version of the burpee you practice. It is one of the best movements for improving both your endurance and your agility. If you are a beginner, try the original version or the knee push-up (knees on the ground for the push-up) version. Start with five or ten in a row, trying not to break the rhythm. You will quickly learn how to pace yourself, and as you progress, work up to doing 40 or 50 without taking a break. After a lot of practice, you just might find yourself doing a 100 in a row. Whichever burpee you choose, make sure you are capable of all the moves, so begin slowly and practice proper form.

If you really want to improve your burpee skills, take the 100-Day Burpee Challenge. The burpee challenge is fairly simple: you start off with one burpee on day one then increase by increments of one each day. The best way to accomplish this challenge is to add it to your cool-down post-workout each day. Below is a chart you can use to check off each day and keep yourself on-task. Make a copy and post it on your refrigerator, in your office, or next to your wall calendar and in 100-days you will be a burpee master, able to take on any obstacle.

100-Day Burpee Challenge

Day 1: 1	Day 26: 26	Day 51: 51	Day 76: 76
Day 2: 2	Day 27: 27	Day 52: 52	Day 77: 77
Day 3: 3	Day 28: 28	Day 53: 53	Day 78: 78
Day 4: 4	Day 29: 29	Day 54: 54	Day 79: 79
Day 5: 5	Day 30: 30	Day 55: 55	Day 80: 80
Day 6: 6	Day 31: 31	Day 56: 56	Day 81: 81
Day 7: 7	Day 32: 32	Day 57: 57	Day 82: 82
Day 8: 8	Day 33: 33	Day 58: 58	Day 83: 83
Day 9: 9	Day 34: 34	Day 59: 59	Day 84: 84
Day 10: 10	Day 35: 35	Day 60: 60	Day 85: 85
Day 11: 11	Day 36: 36	Day 61: 61	Day 86: 86
Day 12: 12	Day 37: 37	Day 62: 62	Day 87: 87
Day 13: 13	Day 38: 38	Day 63: 63	Day 88: 88
Day 14: 14	Day 39: 39	Day 64: 64	Day 89: 89
Day 15: 15	Day 40: 40	Day 65: 65	Day 90: 90
Day 16: 16	Day 41: 41	Day 66: 66	Day 91: 91
Day 17: 17	Day 42: 42	Day 67: 67	Day 92: 92
Day 18: 18	Day 43: 43	Day 68: 68	Day 93: 25
Day 19: 19	Day 44: 44	Day 69: 69	Day 94: 26
Day 20: 20	Day 45: 45	Day 70: 70	Day 95: 95
Day 21: 21	Day 46: 46	Day 71: 71	Day 96: 96
Day 22: 22	Day 47: 47	Day 72: 72	Day 97: 97
Day 23: 23	Day 48: 48	Day 73: 73	Day 98: 98
Day 24: 24	Day 49: 49	Day 74: 74	Day 99: 99
Day 25: 25	Day 50: 50	Day 75: 75	Day 100: 100

SECTION 4

HOW TO GET THROUGH YOUR FIRST RACE

I was completely unprepared for my first obstacle race. I arrived at the race venue in all cotton clothing, looking more like I was ready for a yoga class than an obstacle race. I didn't bring anything to clean the mud off myself after the race, and borrowed a muddy towel from a competitor parked nearby to at least get some mud off of me. I had failed to bring an extra pair of shoes or change of clothing and found myself driving home a muddy mess after the race. This is when I realized the prep for the race can make or break an experience. You don't want your first experience to mirror mine! Luckily, after years of trial and error and some epic fails along the way, my race day kit and plans are dialed in, making each race that much more fun!

On race day, tension is bound to be running high, as you are about to embark on the unknown. With a little preparation and planning you will be able to breeze through the day with the ease of a hardened professional.

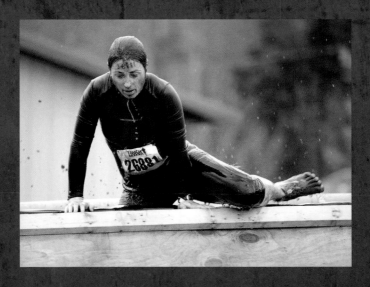

CHAPTER 10

PRE-RACE ESSENTIALS

O ne of the most important things you can do to prepare for your first race starts before you hit the starting line: hydration. The distance of the race determines how far in advance you should start hydrating. For a 5K like the Warrior Dash or Spartan Sprint, a day or two before the race is a great time to hydrate. Plan on cutting any alcohol out of your diet a week before the event, as alcohol will reverse the positive effects of increased water consumption. For the Spartan Beast I spent a full week in advance walking around with a gallon water bottle, which I referred to as my "water

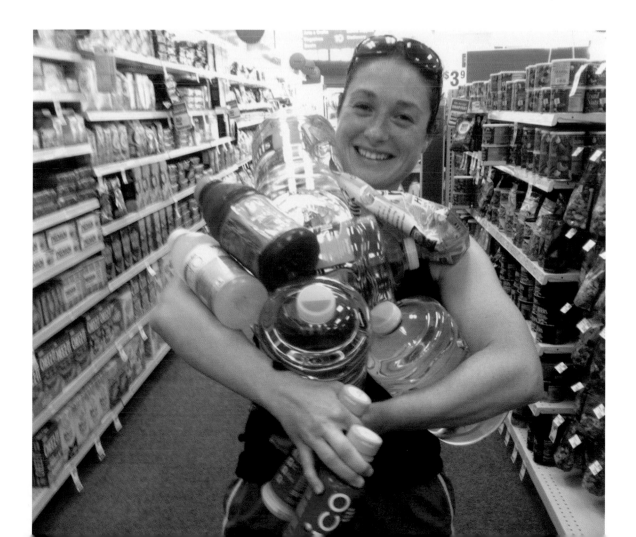

baby." I might have looked funny but I got the proper hydration, which helped me to a podium. On race day itself, make sure you drink enough water, or a mix of half water/half electrolyte drink (e.g., Gatorade) if it's hot outside.

The second most important thing is preparing a well-equipped race day pack. A few extra items packed away have made all the difference for me at races. All race packs should include:

2 – Gallon-sized plastic bags
1 – Tube of sunscreen
1 – Small towel
1 – Beach towel
1 – Travel-size bottle of soap (may sure it's biodegradable)
1 – Full change of clothes (including underwear and socks)
1 – Extra layer of clothing
1 – Pair of flip-flops or extra shoes
2 – Gallon jugs of water
Post-race snacks (calorie-dense)

OK, I know that sounds like a lot of stuff, but each item serves an important purpose. Plastic bags are for your dirty clothes after your race and for your small wet towel. Make sure to apply sunscreen early in the morning and again after you have showered at the race. The first gallon of water is just in case the showers at the race are lousy, so you can just go to your car and use the small towel to wash off with the soap. Most races have gotten better about providing adequate shower facilities, and some even provide soap, but it's always safe to have your own, just in case. The large beach towel will help you change in the parking lot and dry you off.

Here's a little tip I picked up from years of surfing to help you change in a parking lot. First, wrap the beach towel around your body, then pull your wet, muddy underwear off and pull on the clean underwear. Ladies, you can then change your muddy sports bra by holding the wrapped towel, pulling off the wet sports bra and pulling the clean on OVER the towel; then just pull the towel down and you are dressed again!

Double check when packing your race bag to be sure you include the full change of clothes, as this can make the difference between a fun post-race party and a miserable one. Even if it's 100 degrees after a race, you may be susceptible to chills from exerting so much energy, so bring layers. I like to wear flip-flops after a race, but if you need the extra support then pack an extra pair of sneakers.

The second gallon of water is for you to drink up after your race. The free beer that many races give out will not rehydrate you! Many racers have also packed things like bathing suits to shower in, or a baseball cap to keep the sun out.

Race Day Clothing and Shoes

The two most important things on the day of your first race are your clothing and footwear. Obstacle racing will take you through all the elements and across many types of terrain, and you want to make sure that your gear is up for the challenge.

This is the first rule of obstacle racing: DO NOT WEAR COTTON CLOTHING! I have waged a war against cotton in races since I made the rookie mistake in my first race of donning an entire cotton outfit. Why was this a mistake? Cotton is a great fabric, but ill-suited for this task, primarily due to its ability to retain moisture. Since all obstacle races have a mud or water element, a cotton shirt is just going to soak up all the moisture, and once cotton gets wet it loses shape and becomes heavy. I spent much of my first race just pulling up my capris as they sagged further and further off my body. If nothing else, stay away from cotton race clothing; you really don't want to spend a race worrying about losing your pants!

So at this point you might be wondering what you *should* wear. In this case, less is more. I wear as little as possible on race day; my classic outfit is a pair of compression shorts and a bra. When the weather gets cold, it's long compression pants and a compression top. The reasoning behind this minimalist view is that the more clothing you wear, the more mud it will hold, weighing you down. However, many people are not comfortable with this minimalist wardrobe, so when you are starting out look for a form-fitting top in a moisture-wicking fabric. In the warmer months, look for a tank top and in cooler months a long-sleeve. Wicking fabrics are just as key in cool weather races as they are in warmer ones, like the spring Tough Mudder; they help move moisture away from the body to keep your core temperature up when it's cold outside, and in the summer they draw the sweat away from your body. Look for wicking underwear as well; you will be amazed at all the places mud shows up.

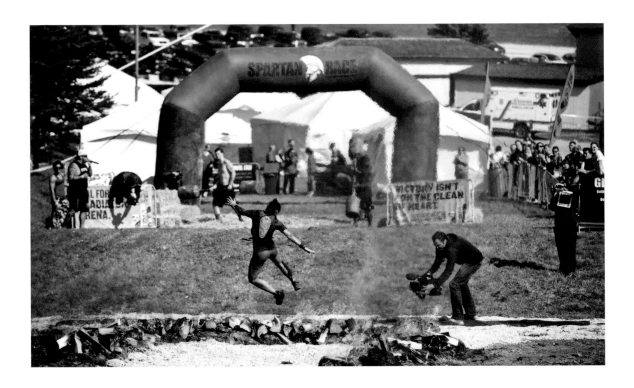

For shorter races (5Ks) I wear shorts, but for longer races, I switch to capris mostly to prevent chafing. Learn where your body's hot spots are so you can lube up before a race. A cheap and effective lubricant is the baby diaper rash cream A&D.

Also, my personal clothing color of choice is black, because it shows no mud or blood from scrapes you sometimes incur along the course, and you never have to worry about stains! Try to stay away from white or other bright colors; they will never be the same after a race; they'll just cause you much aggravation as you try to get stains out.

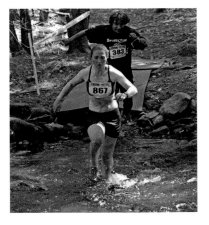

For many people, the idea of donning head-to-toe spandex can be daunting. We can all be a little self-conscious, but when it comes to race day, everyone will be looking at how to get over the obstacles, not at the clothing their competitors are wearing. Once you are wet and muddy, the less clothing you have to move around in, the easier many of the obstacles will be.

Moving on to footwear: I have raced in many different shoes over the last couple of years, so whether you choose a minimalist Vibram Five Fingers (VFF) (done that) or heavy old trail shoes (done that too), make sure you can run in them over varying terrain. Since I started racing in May 2010, I have worn several types of shoes in competition, and each has its advantages. Footwear is an extremely personal subject, and walking

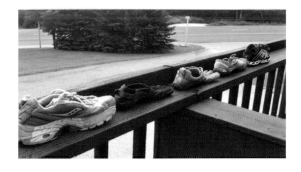

into the shoe store can be daunting with all the choices available today. Unlike sports such as soccer, baseball or football, there isn't one shoe specifically made for obstacle racing. However, many shoes on the market today offer everything you need to have a great race. Through my adventures in shoes I have come up with several key elements to a good obstacle racing shoe.

In my first race I learned why water resistant shoes are not good for obstacle racing. My Solomon Gore-Tex shoes were good at repelling water but when I had to completely submerge my shoe for any period of time, it did a great job of *holding* water. After the first water obstacle, each shoe weighed about 5lbs, which brings me to my second point: swimming in shoes is HARD, and the chunkier the shoe, the harder it is to swim in. Fact. However, traditional trail running shoes have one major advantage: they have grip! When running through mud and scaling walls the tread is a welcome helper. So overall, I learned that you want tread, but don't want a water resistant trail shoe, as the weight of the shoe does matter when your're trying to swim.

My second attempt at a race shoe came on the heels of reading *Born to Run*[23] and, like half of the running world that reads that book, I sped straight over to the nearest store and bought my first pair of Vibram Five Fingers. I thought they would be the answer to the world of running. I quickly learned it takes the body a long time to adjust to this style of running. On

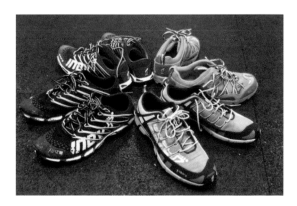

---

23   McDougall, Christopher. *Born to Run: A Hidden Tribe, Superathletes, and the Greatest Race the World Has Never Seen*. Vintage, 2011.

my first obstacle race in Vibrams, I loved the swimming sections; I felt as though I had nothing on my feet, and I loved running in knee-deep mud without the worry of losing a shoe. Unfortunately, they lacked any sort of tread, which made scaling slippery rocks treacherous. I also learned the hard way how easy it is to break a toe or two trail running in them.

I upgraded to another pair of VFFs that had some tread on them and was happy for that. However, I found that when training for longer distances, the damage my feet were incurring on longer and longer trail runs wasn't worth the advantages. I stubbed a lot of toes in the year I ran in them; roots and jagged rocks were like terrorists on a mission to sabotage each run. The more rugged trails I ran the more protection my feet needed from roots and rocks. Overall, I learned from VFFs that minimalist shoes offered the light-weight alternative I was looking for; however, they didn't offer any protection against the unforeseen snares on a trail. They were great in the water, but didn't offer the grip I was looking for. So again, I moved on.

My third attempt at shoes in an effort to stay in the minimalist movement was again inspired by Christopher McDougall's, *Born to Run*. I went searching for a shoe in which I wouldn't constantly be stubbing my toes and I settled on the Merrell Pace Gloves. Yes, I had found the shoe! At least, I thought I had. Yes, this shoe offered the protection against ailing toes and provided the minimalist profile I craved. I liked not having to wear socks with them. But after extensive testing and racing in them, I found that they still were missing the grip. Also, constant movement on the trails with so little padding was not helping my feet and I developed some foot pains.

My most recent venture into the world of shoe testing landed me into the world of Inov-8. At first, I felt like I was selling out going back into a more traditional shoe. In real-ity, the shoe doesn't have much to it but what it does have is important. This shoe offers the minimalist feel and the grip needed for muddy trails and obstacles. It has what can be best described as lugs on the bottom of the shoe, and it's really lightweight. Finally, and perhaps most important, is that this shoe doesn't hold water!

Does this mean that Inov-8 is the only shoe you can race obstacle races in? Absolutely not. However the design of this particular shoe has many of the attributes that make for a great obstacle racing shoe. As of the writing of this book, Inov-8 is the leader in obstacle racing shoes; however, as the sport continues to grow, more and more companies are looking to make obstacle-racing-specific shoes. I am always on the lookout for the best shoe to optimize my race experience. With varying foot widths and sizes it's important to find the shoe that best fits your foot. When picking out your optimum racing shoes look for these five key attributes:

1. Proper Fit
2. Lightweight
3. Good Tread
4. Good Drainage
5. Protection from Rocks/Roots

All that said, the most important thing for race day is to do what you know! Don't try out new shoes the day of a race. Any shoe you are comfortable in can be the best shoe for that day. If you are comfortable, you will be able to run a much better race overall.

Hydration and Nutrition

Once you have your essentials packed, your clothes picked out and your shoes dialed in, there is one more part of the puzzle: your hydration and nutrition plan for race day. Depending on the length of the race and your comfort level, your hydration and nutrition plan will vary. With obstacle course races ranging in distance from 3-mile to over 50-mile races, it is important to have the right plan for the right race. Obstacle course race organizers are notorious for offering minimal aid stations along courses; they are not like your typical road race where every mile is a buffet of food, energy gels, and several choices of water and sports drinks. At most OCRs you will find along the course a few water stations (only one on shorter races), which may include water, a sports drink and maybe a banana. Keeping yourself fueled up while racing is mostly up to you.

In the shorter distance races, carrying additional water and nutrition is not mandatory; however, for your first race it is recommended that you at least carry a gel or a snack in a pocket. Most of the 5K obstacle course races typically take just an hour and a half to complete, but with varying courses and the terrain ever changing, having extra on hand is always helpful. If it is an extremely hot day or you are prone to needing water often, a hydration belt should help you to get from aid station to aid station. A hydration belt is great because it accommodates from one to four small bottles, each typically holding around ten ounces each, of water or a sports drink. The hydration belt offers a lightweight option; you can carry just enough water to get you from aid station to aid station without the extra bulk of a full hydration pack. Most hydration belts also offer a small compartment for a gel or snack. You may have to modify the belt a little to ensure that bottles will not pop out during a barbed wire or swimming obstacle, but normally some string fixes that issue. The hydration belt is the best option for races up to about ten miles or so.

For the long races of over half-marathon distance, you may want to swap out the hydration belt for a hydration pack. A hydration pack offers you the capability to carry more water with you at a time, and gives you more space to carry gels or snacks as well. The belt can also provide space for stashing a headlamp (required by many races if you're starting in the afternoon). The important things to consider when finding a hydration pack are its size and weight. As stated above, there will be aid stations along the course, where you can refill your pack. Therefore, because you will need to carry only half to one liter of water with you at any given time, you do not need a huge hydration pack. The key is to find something that fits close to your body and is comfortable. Try to find fabrics that will repel water and mud, or at least drain well, as your pack will be going through all the obstacles with you.

When shopping for a new pack, look for something small, compact and light. Another option that meets these requirements is a hydration vest, which is a hybrid of a pack and a belt, giving you more space for water but with less bulk than a pack.

The final thing to consider is nutrition. There is a sea of exercise nutrition options, but one of the best for a race is a nutritional gel. Numerous companies make gels of all favors and types; so test some out and see if you like a particular brand. Gels have the advantage of being lightweight, offering you 100 calories at a time. A good rule of thumb is to consume one gel per hour of racing so, depending on the race distance, you may want to stash a couple gels in your belt or pack. Other options, if you dislike the gels, are gummy energy blocks or, for a more natural boost, there is a nut butter company that makes individual 200-calorie packs that can be consumed with the ease of a gel. For races that are longer than a half marathon, I tend to add to my pack a favorite nutritional bar in case I feel weak at any point during the race.

The biggest rule of thumb for attire and nutrition on race day is to not try anything new. Test out a pack in the store before you buy it, or order from a return-friendly company in case the pack doesn't fit well. For your nutrition, try everything out while you are training and preparing for the race. It is important non only that you like the taste of what you are consuming, but also that it sits well in your stomach while you are exercising. These two elements, together with your clothing and shoes, can help you have a successful race.

CHAPTER 11
RACE DAY MORNING

Ok, the time is really here! It's day zero. You trained, your race day pack is set, you have the proper clothing, and you are ready to go! Before you leave the house, print out all registration forms and have them signed before you arrive at the race. If your number is available the night before, then write it down to save some time in registration.

The first thing to do in the morning is to eat a light breakfast. The food you put in your body prior to the race will fuel you through those first couple of miles. It is easy to let your race day jitters get the better of you and lead you to push that important morning meal aside. It is best to keep a banana, apple or quick snack bar in your morning bag, because even on mornings, when jitters are off the charts, I still manage to get down a quick meal. It's also important to make sure that your meal is well-timed so it is not just sitting in your stomach come race time. At one race I astonished my competition when I walked into the race festival area eating a donut before racing. They were shocked by my nutrition choice for the morning, and later laughed and shook their heads as I was on the podium after a second-place finish. For a while we made a joke that donuts made me race faster; in truth, it was not the donut but the dense calories I took in before the race that gave me the energy to race strong that day. If, for example, donuts are the only thing you can manage to eat in the morning, that's still better than nothing, although it's not a pre-race plan I generally advocate. Bottom line, any food on race day morning is better than no food. Find out what works best for your body and work with it.

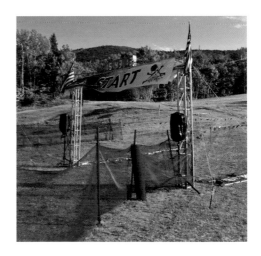

Arrive at the race early; give yourself at least two hours before your heat starts. Arriving early the race venue has a couple advantages; the first is parking. The earlier you arrive the better chance of a good parking space. A good parking space can be like gold after a tough course. Remember to bring some extra cash, as many races charge for parking. The second advantage to arriving early is that you can relax and not feel rushed if lines are long at registration. If night-before registration or pre-race packet pickup is available, do it. It will save you a lot of hassle in the morning. Extra time will allow you to scope out the venue and get a sense of some of the obstacles as, often several obstacles can be seen from the start and finish. Finally, an early arrival gives you a chance to get some last-minute nutrition and a proper warm-up.

Once you have checked in, gotten your number written all over your body (if you like seeing post race pictures do what they say about writing numbers everywhere). A tip to those worried about a permanent marker on their forehead: apply sunscreen first, then write the number; it will come off quickly in the post-race shower. Races today are offering bag check for free or for a nominal fee. Leave any real valuables in your car and put your car keys and ID in your race pack. It's always a good idea to have extra cash in your bag too, for food and other post-race goodies. Other items that are best left at bag check: iPod, sunglasses, baseball caps and wallets. It seems simple but you would be surprised how many people show up to their first race with an iPod or sunglasses; once I even saw a guy with his keys clipped to his shorts! Leave any valuable belongings at home. Music players will get ruined in the water and mud; you will most likely lose your sunglasses in some obstacle, and lock your wallets in the car! I personally stash my wallet out of sight in the car and hide the key.

Warm-Up & The Starting Line

With your bag checked and time to spare, it's now time to warm up for the race. The purpose of the warm-up is more than just getting your muscles loose; it also helps you prepare mentally for the race. If it's your first 5K to 10K distance obstacle race with a goal of finishing, then the warm-up is fairly easy. Start off with a brisk walk for about three to five minutes, then slowly jog for about five minutes, and finally walk again to the starting line. In the starting line give your body a good shake or two, as it will keep everything loose and help you to relax. If you're racing that shorter distance and trying to be competitive, then your warm-up should be more vigorous and, depending on your experience in running, can take up to 45 minutes. Personally, I like to warm up for about

30 to 40 minutes before I race. I like to go for a jog with music on, as it takes my body sometimes a couple miles to warm up. Try different warm-ups in your training so that by race day it becomes automatic.

If your first race is longer than a 10K your warm-up should be less vigorous. Your goal for your first obstacle race should just be to finish. Obstacle races are more taxing than a traditional road or trail run. Your warm-up should just consist of a five to ten-minute brisk walk and jog. Take time after the initial walk or jog to stretch out and feel loose when you are in the starting line. You want to make sure to save your energy for the actual race itself while at the same time staying lose and limber.

For any distances longer than 10K, take a hot shower in the morning and stretch. The shower will help loosen your muscles and wake you up before a race. I personally like to stretch in the shower, and use the time to shake off any last-minute nerves before heading to the race. When you arrive at the race, walk straight to the starting line and conserve energy. The first mile or two will give you the time to warm up.

With your warm-up complete and the starting line in your sights, here are a few pieces of runner's etiquette. If it's your first race and your only goal is to finish, you might not want to push your way to the front with the more experienced competitors. My advice is to stick towards the back of the start so you don't feel pressured when the leaders sprint off and you find yourself moving faster than you trained for. Most obstacle races don't have specific pace sections, so as a rule of thumb for first-timers, hang back in the corral. It will feel that much better when you are passing the leaders on the trail! If you decide to run in a full-on costume, which many obstacle course races encourage, do not line up at the front of the line to start. Guy in the wedding dress, you aren't going for the win, so back off. Let the runners who want to race, race!

As you look around the starting line you are apt to see a lot of people preparing in different ways, but don't let others' actions deter you from your own plan. Just because the guy next to you decided to do 100 burpees before the race, it doesn't make him any faster than you. Or the guy who shotguns a beer with his buddies to show how cool he is on his GoPro video? Let him try to prove what a badass he is. Have a plan and stick with it. Chances are you will probably be passing them after an obstacle or two. In the last few minutes before race time emotions will run high, and the buzz of the crowd will be all around you. Take a few seconds to close your eyes and take a few deep breaths. You have trained, you have prepped, and now comes the fun part: seconds from now the start gun will go off!

CHAPTER 12
THE RACE

In Section 3, you learned all about conquering the obstacles and mentally preparing for the race. Now comes the fun part: the race itself. Try not to get caught in the sprint out of the starting gate, as many of your competitors will do; at this point you know your pace, so stick to it. The obstacles will come and some will be easier than practiced, while others will have you wishing you had put in that extra workout. The most important thing to remember is to have fun and enjoy the experience. The race will challenge you in ways you could never have trained for; this is the unique joy of obstacle racing. The race is much like life, in that you constantly need to adapt and overcome, making the reward of finishing that much sweeter.

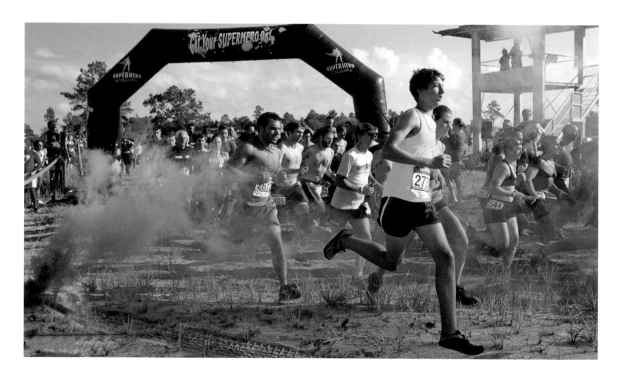

As you stand at the starting line you will feel the excitement. The M/C will start off with a motivating speech or creed to help pump you up. If you are at all worried about the stampede of everyone busting out of the start, then hang back a little and you can start towards the rear. If you are looking for that excitement of the initial 100 yards then elbow further up towards the front. Whichever type of start you prefer, the energy is palpable. Soak in the excitement and be part of it. Don't worry about what the guy next to you is doing; it's all about *your* race. Once the gun,

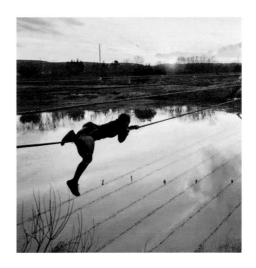

horn, or other starting ritual happens, you are off and it's time to just race.

As you leave the starting line, resist the temptation to go with the herd. People dart out of the start at blistering speed only to slow down and fizzle out a few hundred feet later. Instead of getting sucked into this pattern, start off with a sustainable pace for you. Most obstacle course races include rugged terrain, and a good pace will prove invaluable when a couple miles later you are passing those who were so eager to take off in the first few feet. Save the sprint for the last couple of yards and obstacles.

Many races have the same pattern: they start with a few obstacles followed by a middle section where most of the running is done, and they finish up with a concentration of obstacles at the end of the race. In an untimed mud run, the substance and location of the obstacles can be irrelevant, as it is just about the fun. However, a good pace will have you exploding through the last couple of obstacles and finishing strong. In a race situation, this pattern of obstacles clustered at the end can be part of your race day strategy. Since you pace yourself throughout the whole race, you will have the energy to attack these last obstacles.

At a recent Spartan Race, the last half mile (of a 9-mile race) included a log hop, then a few hundred yards later a swim, followed by the Hercules Hoist, short barbed wire, a slippery wall, a spear throw, a rope climb, the jump over the fire then, finally, the gladiators, followed by the finish line. With more and more races seeking to make the finish fan-friendly, this concentration of obstacles is becoming more and more common. This is where a proper pace at the beginning of the race can give you the edge you need explode though the last half mile. In the case of that particular race, for each missed ob-

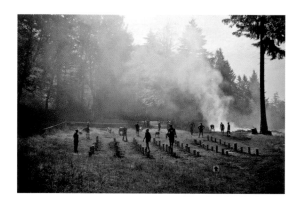

stacle there was a 30-burpee penalty. For even the most elite racers, a fast set of burpees still takes over two minutes, so a few missed obstacles can result in several minutes of difference in a finish time. From a strategic point of view, a lot of time can be made up or lost in the last half mile of the course. In many races I have been able to overtake many athletes who were better runners than I am but couldn't complete those obstacles. And every time you pass someone along the course, it gives you a little boost to go that much faster!

While on the course, an important part of racing is knowing how to properly pass or be passed by other runners. It is common courtesy for racers to step aside for each other in order to let the faster racer pass by. If a racer is barreling up behind you, step aside; he or she may be going for the win. There are three common phrases used by athletes signaling they want to pass, "on your left," "on your right," or simply "behind." Use these phrases when passing fellow competitors and you will sound like a pro. If you are the faster one, please say "thank you" when you pass. I thank each person who moves out of my way; it's a small gesture that goes a long way in the obstacle racing community.

These races are not your average 5K, 10-mile race or even half marathon. If it's your first race, toss out all ideas of what a (for example) 5K time should look like. Some races might take under 30 minutes, others might take an hour for the same distance. The terrain in these races can be gnarly and unforgiving; you maybe running up a mountain or in a state park depending on the race's location, and each race venue is different. Obstacles are meant to slow you down, and they will; it's OK. You will get better at them the more races you do. Use your instincts when confronting an obstacle: if it looks intimidating, take a deep breath then try it again. It took me three attempts to get over one of the walls at the 2011 Vermont Spartan Race Beast, but I still finished the race third for women. Take your time and do it right.

Use the water stations along the race course, even if you are carrying your own hydration. It is important to make sure that you are properly hydrated, especially through the longer races where a few seconds of rehydrating might give you the energy to push past your competitors at the end. If the aid station has a banana or other food, it might be a good idea to eat as well. If you are carrying your own hydration and nutrition, use the stations to keep your bottles full of water or, if it's particularly hot, dump a cup or two over your head to cool down. At the end of the race, getting your hair wet will be the least of your worries, and for the moment it can offer a nice reprieve, especially in desert races. Even in my shortest races a well-timed aid station can mean the difference between a podium finish and dropping out of the top ten, or sometimes the difference between finishing and not finishing a race.

In 2011, Hobie Call, the famed Spartan Racer and arguably the world's best obstacle course racer, lost his first race in Vermont at the inaugural Spartan Race Beast. He underestimated the course, bonked[24] along the way, and finished the race barely in the top ten. During the race he bonked so hard that he struggled to get back to an aid station, take in some nutrition, and then continue onward to finish the race. Even the most seasoned athlete in the sport admits that he underestimated that race. As Hobie found out that August day in 2011, never underestimate a course, use the aid stations, and make sure you have a plan as you head in to the race.

Most importantly, run your own race; results ultimately don't matter as long as you know you pushed hard. Have a great time and meet new people who share your interest in this amazing sport. If you are lucky enough to have a group to race with, then cheer each other on. If competing is your goal, maybe you can take home a cool sword[25] at the end of the day! Above all, it's about you and finding out a little bit more about yourself and earning some impressive scrapes and bruises to show off at work on Monday!

As you cross the finish line, if you're anything like me, you will feel a sense of emotion not experienced in most daily activities. As they place the medal around your neck, you will know that your hard work and dedication paid off. Go enjoy your free drink and start downing that gallon of water. Talk with other racers about the course at the finish line.

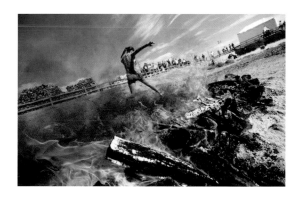

---

24 Also known as "Hitting the Wall." A bonk is when you have depleted the glycogen stores in your liver and muscles, causing a sudden fatigue and loss of energy to set in. Many times carbohydrate-filled food or drink can remedy the situation. The term originates in cycling and has transcended sports to become a general term.
25 Winner's prize at the Spartan Race from 2010 – 2012.

CHAPTER 13
STORIES FROM THE COURSE

Every obstacle course racing champion started somewhere; no one wakes up one day to suddenly break world records. Each racer has his or her own story, journey and reasons why OCR is their sport of choice. The following stories are from a variety of racers. Some often find themselves on the podium while others have used OCR to help change their lives and, in one case, regain a life. The stories below are diverse, offering tips for race day and strategies that have helped achieve goals at all levels.

Shelley Koenig

Shelley is a chemistry teacher and mother of two. She had always been one to favor the outdoors but obstacle course racing opened a new door in her life. She has not only tackled and succeeded in Tough Mudders, Spartan Races, and World's Toughest Mudder, but she is also the 2012 Female summer Death Race winner. She is a tough Mainer who

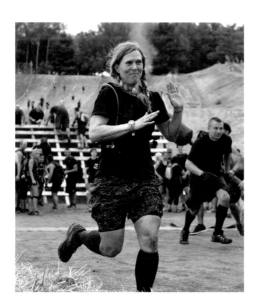

always races with a smile on her face. In her own words, here are Shelley's tips for the new racer:

By no means would I describe myself as a pro in the obstacle racing circuit. In fact, I am not sure that I could fairly describe myself as a pro at anything. Some days I am wildly successful, some days are utter failures, but most days are a mix. In the last few years, I have been fortunate enough to become part of the obstacle racing community, a community of extraordinary people who have forced me to challenge my own weaknesses, helped me see my strengths, and accepted me without judgment. I have gained a sense of belonging amongst friends simply through shared experiences. This community has looked out for me on a journey to find myself. On one occasion, I was (literally) picked up off the ground by a total stranger who helped me press on when I thought quitting was my only option. On another occasion, friends of only a few short hours shared their food and water with me when I was unprepared. I have learned much from the people in this amazing community. I have learned that the approach to every race, every training session, and every moment in our lives really ought to be the same.

So, here is my attempt to impart a top-five list of things this community has taught me for those who are thinking about giving their first OCR event a shot.

1. Remove "can't" from your vocabulary. Failure is only how you define it. If you are paralyzed by a fear of failing, you deny yourself opportunity for growth. We all fail to meet our goals sometimes; this is part of achieving success.

2. Be open to celebrating the camaraderie of obstacle racing. People will offer you their hands, backs, shoulders or whatever it takes to help you complete obstacles. As you become more experienced, you can return the favor to others.

3. Embrace burpees. Guaranteed: somewhere you will be asked to do them; you might as well enjoy them.

4. Don't steer around the things that scare you. Go over them. Go through them. They have nothing on the strength inside you.

5. Don't take yourself too seriously. I used to train meticulously. I calculated miles, weights, and max heart rate. I worried about it all. Racing in my first Tough Mudder, I glanced over at my training partner and noticed that she had mud between her teeth and her long blonde hair was dyed blue and resembled tangled seaweed. I told her she looked ridiculous. She poked me and replied, "What do you think you look like?" We giggled the rest of the way. Enjoy every moment of the experience. Before you know it, you'll be looking for the next one.

In short, the joy is in the process. Savor the small victories. Each small victory slowly will erode the notion of the unattainable and provide a foothold for the next step. Embrace your failures. Only in failure are we forced to define our weaknesses. Realize that life is the race, a race where victory isn't defined by the successes of someone else; rather, it is defined by what you do with the miles that lie before you. Do you curse the miles ahead, focus on discomfort, and focus solely on reaching the end? Every race has its end, whether we know where it is or not. Savor each step, appreciate the path ahead and know that the strength to confront challenges already lies within you.

Chris Rutz

Some find local 5Ks to run each weekend; Chris Rutz follows the obstacle racing circuit. When he decides to do something, he does it 100 percent. He is a regular at the Spartan Race series, taking part in more races in 2012 than any other person in the world. Not only did he race; he also finished the end of the season ranked third in the world. Not bad for a guy who often refers to himself as the "masters" racer, as his license shows his age as over 40. He has taught the young ones a thing or two in the last couple of

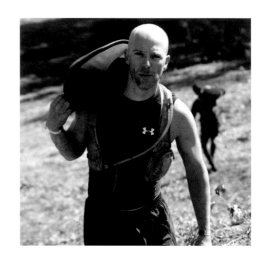

years; it's clearly not just a sport for the young. Here are Chris's tips for success:

So, you want to run your first obstacle race? Maybe you have seen pictures of the ultra-fit men and women plastered on Facebook and the race websites, or maybe a friend or a family member took you to a race. Perhaps you are a runner who has heard of these "mud runs." You have decided to step up and register for your first race. What next? What do you do now?

My three step plan for finishing your first obstacle race:
- Stay Calm
- Be Anxious
- Be Eager

Stay Calm:

Literally hundreds of thousands of people have done an obstacle race, perhaps even millions. They are people from all walks of life, all sorts of athletic or non-athletic backgrounds.

There are moms, dads, grandmothers, grandfathers and kids. There are people who weighed 200, 300, 400 pounds. There are people without legs, arms or both. If they can run an obstacle race, so can you.

Be Anxious:

Now that you are calm, it is time to make yourself nervous. Sure, you could go into the race without any training and walk much of the course and skip the obstacles but that would quite literally be "a walk in the park." If that is what you want, go for it. On the other hand, these are not easy events if you want to complete every obstacle and the entire course. You need to do some training. Running. Yes, running; I know you do not like running. Keep at it; you will grow to love it. Burpees; same thing. You know what a burpee is right? Strongly recommend burpees. Not just because some races make you do them, but because they are a great overall exercise. Push-ups, pull-ups, squats, mountain climbers. Pick up something, anything and carry it for a while. Put it down, pick it back up. You need to get in shape for this thing and you need to get in shape for life. You do want a life, right?

Be Eager:

Okay, I have convinced you that you can do it. You have trained—maybe a lot, maybe a little. Whatever you did or did not do, today is the day. Get to the start line and be eager, not anxious. Eager to run your first obstacle race, eager to climb that first wall, eager to get that finisher medal, eager to get that t-shirt. Most importantly, be eager to call yourself an Obstacle Racer. Get out there and get your feet wet, get a few scratches, get some dirt in your face. It is so worth it!

Juliana Sproles

Juliana and I briefly met in 2011 at World's Toughest Mudder, she had just won the women's race. I was eager to meet this woman who was able to brave the hypothermic temperatures and be one of only two women to finish the race. However, it wasn't until 2012 that we got to know each other. Juliana has an unwavering passion for anything she does and gives

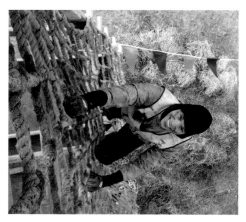

it everything she has once she gets started. Below is her story from the 2011 World's Toughest Mudder:

Again and again, I was slipping and sinking up to my ears in icy, dark, murky, muddy water, breaking through sheets of ice as I went. I had become tired of trying to carefully move myself forward through a series of very long, deep, slimy mud pits only to fall up to my eyeballs into unknown sinkholes every few steps. There was simply no way to gracefully walk across this particular "Mud Mile," scramble up the embankment, climb up and over an 8-foot wall and ease back down into the muck just to do it all over again, five, six or seven times to the far side of the pit. I needed a new strategy.

"Thirty-two is better than twenty-seven." I kept saying it over and over. I was there. I was deep in the first-ever 24-hour obstacle course known as the "World's Toughest Mudder." I was literally freezing but I absolutely would not let myself admit it. I would not allow myself to shiver nor shake for even an instant. I knew that if I did, it would all be over. Instead, I continually kept asking everyone around me what the air temperature was and I developed a mantra (several of them, actually) to help me survive the madness. In my mind, I thought that every time I entered the water, if it wasn't frozen, it must be at least 32 degrees. On the other hand, the air temperature was dropping every time I asked, and the wind chill was cutting through my Mylar, nylon, neoprene and wool layers like a knife. There was nowhere to hide. I decided that-under the water was the best place to be I could relax my body, rest a minute and shield it from the fierce and unrelenting wind that kept stealing away my body heat. So I kept saying it over and over, "32 is better than 27." It didn't matter if this made any sense or not; it worked for me. And since we had so many water obstacles to navigate, I got to practice my mantra consistently throughout the race, and I swam through or skimmed across as many water obstacles as I could.

How did I get to this place? What was I doing here? And why? Why was I running through mud, around in circles like a hamster on an artic ice wheel? On a regular basis, I ask myself and am asked these questions. Only now, it seems, everyone is doing it and everyone has the answers. They truly "get it." So many athletes and weekend warriors have discovered the thrill of navigating great physical obstacles on muddy courses all over the globe. We pay to play in mud and come home with great stories. We share our triumphs, our trials and tribulations. We are elated. We connect with our comrades and we are happy. We are human. We are truly alive.

After 30 years of running and 24 years of age-group triathlons I was bored, it was time for something new. My friend, Brooke, came home from a weekend away and described this new event she volunteered for where "people run through mud and fire!" I asked about the fire, and she said, "It's really just little fire." I was intrigued and we decided as a team to try it out the next time Tough Mudder came to town. I agreed to this adventure with much trepidation, skepticism and doubt. Having a tendency toward claustrophobia, I was not at all excited to enter cold, dark, wet tunnels and other small, dark cramped places, nor to be electrocuted, but I went along with the plan anyway, with my teammates by my side.

It was May 2011, Memorial Day Weekend at Snow Valley, a ski resort in Southern California. The forecast called for freezing rain and harsh wind chill. We hadn't really believed the forecast, but my two teammates and I found ourselves shivering in a near-hypothermic state on top of a deserted ski run in the middle of our very first Tough Mudder challenge. We had to make a decision—and fast. Any heat we had managed to trap within our less than adequate layers of clothing had just been stripped away after we emerged from full submersion into what was then known as Chernobyl—a gigantic tractor-trailer-long ice bath. After that, we did manage to make our way straight up the side of a mountain in spite of the cold and wind chill cutting through us sideways. I wrapped a piece of discarded Mylar around my head like a turban, convinced myself I was warm and carried on. It was one of the hardest things I've ever done, but we finished our very first Tough Mudder under some of the harshest conditions and brought home several war stories from our battle with ice, wind, electricity, broken noses and, more importantly, with ourselves. On the drive home, I exclaimed to my teammates, "I know how to go 24 hours. I am going to World's Toughest Mudder." Right then and there, I submitted our team time via email and cemented the idea in my mind.

Even though they were invited, my teammates declined to join me in my quest for World's Toughest Mudder. I was excited about it anyway and set out to prepare for it. I recruited help from my outdoor exercise group and we completed several kinds of workouts together. I went through quite a mental process and, finally, I convinced myself that I was capable of winning WTM 2011. I arrived in Englishtown, NJ and sought out other female competitors, but couldn't locate any until just before the start. About 900 of us took off at the starting line. Twenty-four hours and five minutes later two of us crossed together. Junyong Pak and I agreed to run across the line at the same time even though he had completed one lap more than I did. This is how I won World's Toughest Mudder.

I had no idea what it would feel like to stand upon a stage and receive a $10,000 prize for doing something as crazy as navigating cargo nets, mud, barbed wire, electricity, ice, physical exhaustion and mental demons all day and all night under such frigid conditions, with no sleep and minimal gear to keep warm. It was a true test of the human spirit. Even though it was definitely a race, we helped one another and we all came away with a sense of pride in how much we were able to endure. It didn't matter how many laps we completed. We were there. We put World's Toughest Mudder 2011 into the history books. My summary was this, "It was cold. It was hard. It was good. It was great. It was amazing!" And, yes, I would do it all over again.

Andi Hardy

I first met Andi in Spring 2012. She had recently won her first race and was emerging onto the race scene. In 2012, racing for Andi became much more than just about the medals and the trophies. We all saw a change in Andi: she seemed to blossom during the year, gaining confidence at each race. She made new friends and traveled around the country (mostly in her little red late 80s BMW). Wearing her trademark lime green, this woman literally transformed before our eyes and the eyes of the OCR world. Here is Andi's story:

At 42 years old my life as I knew it was changing quickly before my own eyes. My business went under, my daughter left for college, my marriage fell apart, and I was moving out of the dream house I had built on a beautiful mountain lake. What could I do?

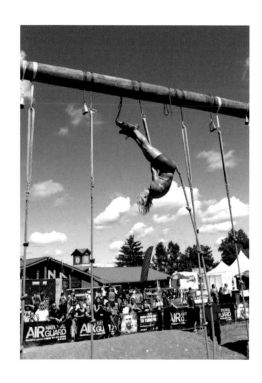

I was forced to try new things in life, so why not try something new in the lines of fitness as well? After training three days a week for a sprint triathlon I realized that I could run three miles. I had only intended to walk the three miles of the tri, but found that the competitor in me could not simply walk. Two weeks later I found myself winning my age division in a 3-mile obstacle mud run. Two weeks of running and I placed better than 128 women my age. Hmmm, what if I actually trained? What could I accomplish?

I heard about the Spartan Race, an obstacle course race, and signed up immediately. It was almost five months away, but that would give me time to train. I trained every day, taking rest days when really needed. I felt great physically and mentally. All of the stresses of life were much more manageable with fitness now a big part of my life.

I won't say I wasn't a nervous wreck for that first race. The competitor in me put the pressure on to do as well as I could, and perhaps place at the top of my age division. The athlete in me was ready for a challenge unlike any I had ever faced. But, like many, I feared the unknown. I questioned whether I would even be able to finish, much less do well.

I started at the very back of the pack and hoped for the best. Little by little I passed competitor after competitor. I watched those ahead of me complete obstacles, and somehow I managed to learn really quickly what to do. I also learned quickly what happens when you miss an obstacle (in my case the spear throw): 30 burpees really fast.

I pushed myself, I dug deep, I yelled words of encouragement to others because it also helped me. I somehow made it to the finish line, and the pictures show I was even smiling!!

What an accomplishment! I was elated and totally driven. Little did I know it that day, but I would be repeating that feat over twenty more times in the upcoming nine months. Trying something new turned into a new love, a new passion, and a new lifestyle. Don't be afraid of the unknown; you never know, it could be your next step in life.

Chris Davis

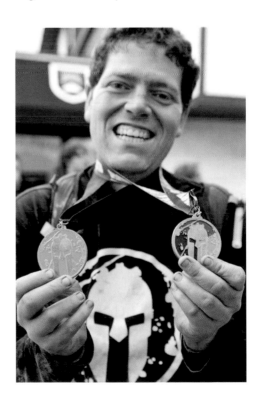

I first met Chris Davis while participating in the Spartan Race Coaching Certification in spring 2012. Chris came to Vermont to train under Spartan staff to help him get in shape for the Vermont Beast to be held in September. Chris at his heaviest had weighed 696 pounds, and when we met he was just under 400 pounds. He had competed in the Spartan Race Sprint in Georgia before coming to Vermont. I had the good fortune to work with him as his trainer for the last two months of his program and watch him slim down to 265 pounds by race day thanks to diet, exercise and a lot of hard work. This is his story:

I can remember it as if it were yesterday. It was 3 a.m. and I was about to head out for the biggest challenge of my life: I was going to take on Killington Mountain to complete my first Spartan Beast. But this was no regular Spartan Beast—it was the Vermont Beast. The Vermont Beast is the Championship Race because it is one of the toughest, steepest, and most feared races in the Spartan Series. After getting into the car, I had a moment when I asked myself what in the world had I gotten myself into. Five months ago, I had a similar incident when I was pulling into the parking lot of my first Spartan Race in Georgia. I could not help but laugh; that race was only four miles, and it almost killed me. Now, I was off to do a 15-mile race. A few minutes later, we pulled into Dirt in Your Skirt HQ, and Forest Call joined me. A few months earlier he had heard about what I was trying to do, and he had offered to be by my side and film the whole race with me. I cannot tell you how much it meant to me to have someone by my side as I was going through this adventure. If there is one thing I have learned over the last year is that when you are trying to do anything outside of your comfort zone, it really helps to have someone there with you. If you do not have someone with you before you head out, find someone while you are on your adventure, and team up. I cannot tell you how many times I have wanted to quit, but kept going because I was with someone else, and I was not going to leave them alone.

It was almost 4 a.m. before everyone arrived at Killington Mountain. You could see your breath, and I swear there was a thin sheet of ice on the water in the obstacles. After the first hour or so, everything just felt surreal. It no longer felt like a race; it turned into another training day with Joe Desena (Spartan Race founder) as he led us up the mountain. I have never been as happy to see the sun as I was that day. The funny thing was, as the sun started to rise the situation changed from being on a hike back to be being in the Spartan Race. I saw the festival area start to fill with people, the music started up, and we started to back towards the festival and the 4-mile checkpoint. That was the first moment when I started to realize that I was in trouble.

My original plan was to complete two laps, and come home with the Ultra Beast. But it was almost 8 a.m. when we reached the 4-mile cut checkpoint, so did the mental math and realized I had another 20+ hours of race course ahead of me. That had me worried, but I pushed it out of my mind and kept on going. I had to keep focusing on the next obstacle or the next hill. I could not afford to think about everything I still had ahead of me, because I knew that if I did that I'd completely freak out. So I kept my focus on whatever was next, until famed obstacle racer Hobie Call came running past me. It was good to see him go by, but I knew that he had completed the same amount of the course in an hour as had taken me five hours. That is when I started to doubt that I'd be able to complete the race. I was so cold, tired, and now getting sore, and being lapped by people that started the race over four hours after I did. That was when I had to remind myself that I was not racing them—I was there to challenge myself, to see how far I could push myself, to see how far I had come since my first Spartan Race. That that was all that it took to get past that bout of doubt.

As each additional racer passed me, I felt stronger and stronger. It was like I had started to feed off their energy, and it was just what I needed to keep me going. Being around so many other racers was an incredible feeling; even the bad times didn't seem so bad because we were all in it together.

That feeling stayed with me until the climb up Bear Mountain. The climb for me started late in the afternoon, after I had been on the course for about ten hours. I was starting to run out of strength, and I was finding myself taking a lot of breaks. The Bear Mountain climb was one of the longest, most brain-teasing climbs because it was switchback after switchback, up the side of the mountain, in thick woods. This went on for what seemed like forever. There were so many times during this part of the race that I wanted to quit, but I knew there was no way off the side of the mountain, and I would need to keep going to reach a safe place to be rescued. I really felt I was in trouble, and this is the point where having a friend by your side becomes so important. I knew that if I got into trouble he would get help. So I pushed on further than I ever thought possible. Finally we made it to the top, and I'm not going to lie—I wanted to pass out and die. That was when I bumped into my friend Kaitlyn Hummel on the course. We sat there and talked about what we had just survived, and started to laugh about it all. It was just what I needed to regroup and continue on.

Everything was going good again, until the log hop. I was doing fine until the last log. It was just so far away.... I knew that as long as I touched it I was OK. I took a giant step, touched it, then fell off. I hit the ground hard—*very* hard. I hit so hard that I could not get up; I could not even move. I had ringing in my ears. A few seconds later, I was able to start moving again, but my left leg felt like it was on fire. I checked it out and found no obvious injuries, so I tried to get up and walk. That was when the real pain started; luckily, so did the adrenaline. All of a sudden the pain didn't seem so bad. So on I went—limping, but moving forward. I knew any plans I had for completing the Ultra Beast were gone. Now my goal was just to survive the Beast. I was near the end and I was not going to quit, so I dug in deep, and just focused on one step at a time. That was all that I could handle. I was in survival mode for the rest of the race.

I learned so many things about myself in this race. The first, and for me the most important discovery, was that I can push myself to try things that I think are impossible. Another key thing I learned is that I should never be afraid to ask for help: I am not alone; there is someone else going through the same thing I am, and together we are stronger. Lesson three: sometimes you have to stop thinking about the big picture, and just focus on one step at a time. Lastly, I learned that challenging yourself to do the impossible changes your life. You start to ask yourself, "If I can climb a mountain, what else can I do?"

SECTION 5

WHAT'S NEXT?

I still remember the feeling after completing my first obstacle course race in 2010 that something had changed within me. I had only signed up to do the Spartan Race on a whim, since it was close to home. I wasn't a runner, I had no specific goals, and I certainly had no preconceived notions of what lay ahead. All I knew on that day was I wanted more. I had already started on a path to a healthier, more balanced life, but it was after crossing that finish line that something truly clicked for me. I stood at the finish line muddy and wet, but satisfied in a way I hadn't felt for a long time.

I got home that night, clothing still a muddy mess, and started to frantically search the web for more of these "obstacle course races." I would go on that summer to compete in two more races, another Spartan Race and a War-

rior Dash. I remembered seeing Tough Mudder and thinking I would never be able to compete in a race like that. This was the first of many times that I would think there was is no way I could do a particular race or challenge, only to find myself months or years later doing that very thing.

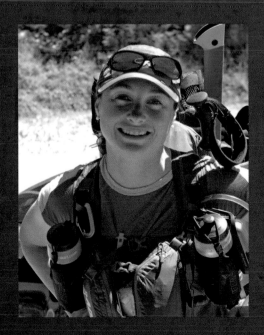

When I started this journey in 2010 I had never been a "runner" of any kind, and certainly not a distance runner. A few years later I find myself a new person; I am now an obstacle course racer, an Ultra-marathoner, a Death Racer, and an overall a competitive athlete at levels I had never dreamed of. In winter 2013, I took on another race that would again challenge all that

I knew. Not only was the Fuego y Agua Survival Run a jungle obstacle course race set on an island in Nicaragua formed by two volcanoes, it also was a 75-kilometer (nearly 50-mile) race in which I would carry a live chicken for five miles, run handcuffed, carry 40 pounds of firewood on my back, drag 60-pound logs, dig through sand, carry a 20-foot bamboo pole up a volcano, and climb a tree up over 25 feet in the air. Somehow I managed to do all of these things while sustaining myself with water and nutrition for long stretches of time and keeping a smile on my face. Had you spoken to my former self in May 2010, she would have laughed at the idea of my even thinking about such a race. But here I am just a few short years later, not only competing with the best in the sport but holding my own alongside them. I continue to amaze myself when I look back and think about the things I have done or attempted to do in the last couple of years. Whether your own path takes you to more racing or just to a new direction in life, remember to never say "never" and stay open to all possibilities; you will be amazed at what you are capable of.

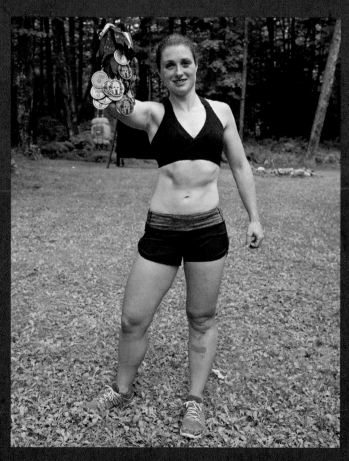

CHAPTER 14

POST-RACE EXPECTATIONS & ADVICE

Y ou finished your first race! You washed the mud off your body, changed back into clothing that isn't lycra-based or sopping wet. You may or may not have slept wearing the medal in bed last night. It's perfectly normal to never want to take it off. Obstacle course racing gives you a thrill that no road race can ever bring. You might even wear the medal to work or hang it up in your workspace. It seems life is getting back to normal, albeit with a few scrapes and bruises adorning your body. But something feels different: you feel changed!

It's Monday morning back at work. The scrapes are covered up and you are feeling a bit of the Clarke Kent/Superman complex. Over the weekend you felt alive, got dirty,

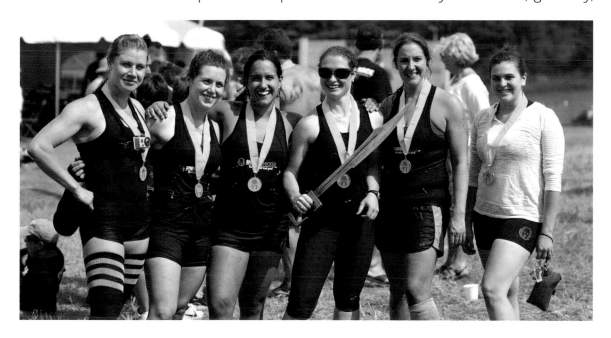

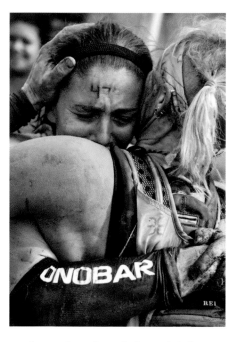

and may have had a life-changing moment on the course. I know that the first time I climbed over an 8-foot wall unassisted was pretty special, as was finally conquering the rope traverse. We find ourselves a bit changed but our surroundings are the same. The clock still ticks on the wall as we count down the hours until the workday is over. The coffee is still a little burned in the pot, and the phone rings while emails pour in. Life goes on whether we are ready for it or not.

You try to recount the weekend stories to your co-workers and are lucky to get more than a "you're crazy" or "you did this for fun (raised eyebrow)?" I find the more enthusiastic I am about a story, the more people think I am absolutely crazy. You just smile and nod, sad they didn't experience the same exhilaration over the weekend that you did. They will never fully understand until they do it. Trust me: this is all NORMAL!

You will find yourself seeking out races in other locations during the downtime of your workday and trying to work out family and life events around races. You are becoming an obstacle racer! You find yourself running to Facebook during the day to check out what your friends posted about the race. Did you see their bruises? Yes, I already claimed my results on athlinks.com. You may compulsively keep hitting the refresh button on the race photographer's website to see what photos came up from the past weekend. No, the pictures are not all up on Monday morning from the race on Saturday. All these things often came into my head during that first day back at work; it was always a hard day to focus. Also, the longer the race or more intense the experience, the harder it is to just sweep it under the rug and go about the day. So what about work? You probably aren't going to want to be back in the grind right away. But instead of using up sick days to recount the weekend's activities, there are a few ways to make this readjustment easier.

1. RIDE THE POST-RACE HIGH

It's fun! Tell the stories, wear the medal, rep those bruises. You accomplished a great task over the weekend, so own it! Expect to feel the runner's high; you probably feel like a new person.

2. PREP FOR THE CRASH

The longer the race, the harder the crash. You are amped up after the race but everything around you is the same. You want to yell to the rafters about this transcendent experience you had but that no one else seems to understand. Other racers understand; if you can, talk with them when you start to feel the flat line. Don't let the blues weigh you down. Some find a new race and sign up to work towards a new goal.

After World's Toughest Mudder in 2011, I had a hard time adjusting back to normal life for a couple days. I was combating extreme fatigue and minor hypothermia, and had just pushed further and harder than I had ever gone before. I was a wreck as I sat at the front desk of the school I worked in at the time. I was definitely a different type of greeter for people that week, as my skin had an almost greenish tint to it. Not only was my physical appearance different, I felt an overall malaise. Fortunately, a friend and former multi-day adventure racer really helped me through with some supportive words. We had a brief conversation via Facebook the day I returned to normal life. I felt a little lost back in the world outside the race, and his words to me that day still rank as the best I have ever heard after a race. If you are feeling down seek out some racing friends. They will help you through. They don't need to be obstacle course racers, either, as most types of racers understand this malaise and are willing to talk though it.

3. EASE BACK INTO WORK

At 8:00 a.m. you sit at your desk looking at a long list of emails or stack of to-do's. It all doesn't seem to matter as much anymore. Take the day slowly. Take one email at a time and let yourself take the extra time, if you can. Otherwise, try to resist the temptation to stare at race photos all day.

4. TAKE CARE OF YOUR BODY

Clean your wounds; you should have already done this by now, but maybe you were just too sore or tired. Monday night in the shower, really clean out all those scrapes and cuts. If you have a bathtub, take a long Epsom salt soak. Epsom salt will help with the soreness and bruises. If you have blisters, take care of them; I like to soak my feet in some iodine diluted water to kill any bacteria that may be in an open blister or lingering on my feet. Oh, and if you ran A LOT, be prepared to lose a few toenails. In general, take care of your body; if this was your first race you will be sore in places you didn't know existed! Take the day off and rest your body from any crazy exercise.

5. HYDRATE

Keep a bottle of water with you all day and rehydrate after the weekend. Chances are that between the race and the after-party, you dehydrated your body. Take that office time to sit, relax and sip some cool water all day long.

6. GEAR

Don't let your wet and muddy gear just sit in a bag because it's too dirty to deal with. I have done this and the results haven't been good! Some of my clothing years later still smells like that New Jersey water from World's Toughest Mudder, no matter how many times I wash it. If you can dry out your clothing before putting it in the washer, do it. Try to knock as much dried mud off your clothing and socks beforehand. The less dirt on your clothing prior to it going in the wash, the less likely you are to find a dirt ring at the bottom of the washer. You may even wish to use a garden hose to rinse off the clothing before you pop it into the washer. After the 2012 Spartan Race in the Mid-West I found myself at the car wash rinsing the mud off my clothing after I'd let it sit around for a few days. This was an extreme case! A final tip to help really get your clothing clean is to wash your race clothing twice, the first time with a half-cup of Pine Sol then again with your regular detergent. The Pine Sol will greatly help get the dirt out without damaging your race gear. You will have fresh clean clothing ready for your next race.

Lastly, just enjoy the day and the moment. You accomplished something great and the accomplishment was fully yours. People will never understand what they haven't done and you will never fully be able to explain it. Once those race photos are out you can print them, put them up in your workspace, then wait for your co-workers to *want* to hear the stories. Next time, if the stories are good enough, they might just be joining you at the starting line.

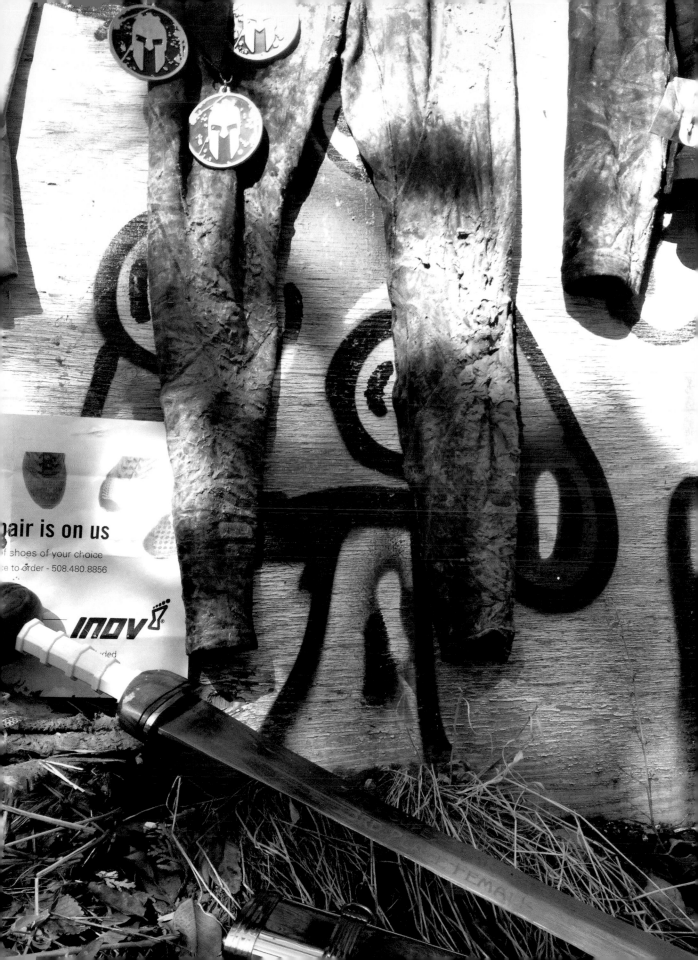

CHAPTER 15

RECOVERY

The most predictable thing about any mud run or obstacle race is that, the next day, you will be sore, and the day after that, even more so. Obstacle course racing has a way of not only making your typical running muscles sore, but also leads to soreness in places that seem unrelated. The oddest place I have ever been sore was my knuckles. It wasn't until I analyzed the race that the source of the soreness revealed itself: the bucket carry. I had locked my knuckles under the bucket during the race and a day later had to wonder whether it was the early onset of arthritis or just soreness (thankfully I was only sore)! Fingers are not the only odd place that post-race soreness sets in. Two days after the race you will be learning more about obscure muscles you never knew you had. Knowing this going into a race allows you to appropriately plan your recovery time.

Proper recovery techniques can have a huge effect on the amount of time it takes for those aches to go away so you can get ready for your next adventure. The very first thing is to take a day or two off from exercise. A good ice bath post-race can help ease the initial soreness. Ice baths are a form of cryotherapy ("cold therapy") which constricts blood vessels and decreases metabolic activity. This in turn helps to reduce swelling and tissue breakdown. It can greatly aid in decreasing the appearance of those black and blue bruises post-race. Once the skin is no longer in contact with the cold source, the underlying tissues warm up, causing a return of faster blood flow, which helps return the byproducts of cellular breakdown to the lymph system for efficient recycling by the body. Ice baths not only suppress inflammation, but also help to flush harmful metabolic debris out of your muscles. In any case, after a mud run or obstacle course race, an ice bath can be essential to your recovery. If you are into the exact science, when making your ice bath the temperature should range from 50 to 59 degrees (it does not need to be Arctic temperature), and you should stay in for 10 to 20 minutes. I have a friend who has a cold stream near his house and instead of an ice bath he just spends time in the stream with a good book. In addition to an ice bath and some stretching, it is very important to let your body rest and recover.

Take the time to let your body regenerate just as you did during training. A race puts a huge amount of impact on the body, and even for the most seasoned athlete a good recovery day post-race is important. After your first race it is particularly important to take the first day off as a complete rest day, eat lots of healthy food, drink lots of water and, as stated earlier, really make sure all dirt is gone from your body (check behind your ears). Take the time to catch up on a good television show, read a book, or relax around the house. For the active person, this complete recovery can be hard, but you will probably savor the idea of doing nothing after your first race.

On the second day of post-race recovery, begin what's referred to as "active recovery." This is where you are moving around again, working your muscles but not taxing them. This might entail a walk around the neighborhood or a short trail run at a comfortable talking pace. Others find that spinning on a stationary bike is a great low impact way to get the blood moving and break up the lactic acid that builds up in muscles after a race. Lactic acid building is, in simplest terms, something that occurs after a strenuous workout from the body breaking down different compounds to create energy. Whichever is the best medium for you, it's important to move around even though you are most likely even more sore than the day before. After about 20 to 30 minutes of moving around, it is important to get a quality stretch. There are two forms of stretching—active and passive—that can be used as part of an active recovery. The following section details active stretching, as it is the best form of stretching for recovery.

Active Stretching

Active stretching involves movement-based stretches (think walking around the room while stretching out). These can be done with little or no warm-up, are important to recovery and can even be incorporated into your training routine. To execute an active stretch, you will need about 20 meters of space. A local track is an excellent place for a recovery workout, as you can warm-up with a few loops around the track then use the soccer or football field to do the active stretching. A standard set of exercises that can easily be executed are outlined in the pages that follow. As with all other forms of exercise, when engaging in an active stretch you should start off slowly; as the muscles warm up, the stretching can become deeper and positions be held longer. It is very important not to try to do too much too quickly. Here are a few examples from one active recovery stretch sequence; each one is meant to be done on a field or in a gym. You should complete each one down and back about 10 to 15 meters.

Opposite Hand Opposite Foot: As you step forward, kick one foot up into the air to meet opposite side's outstretched hand. Then step forward and switch the hand and foot. As you continue to move forward, you will be able to kick your foot up higher to reach the hand and will be able to move faster.

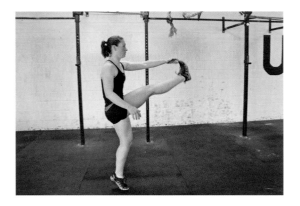 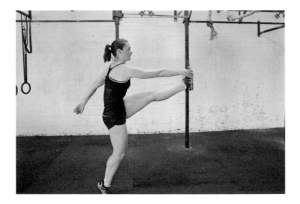

Hugging Knees: As you step forward, balance on one foot, pulling the other leg towards your chest and grasping your shin with your arms. Hug the knee close to you. Switch feet. Once you have mastered your balance, roll up onto the toes of your "standing foot" for a deeper stretch.

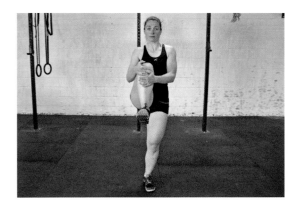 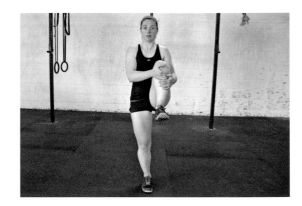

Yoga Twists: Hold your hands in a prayer position, palms pressed together. Step forward with your right foot into a lunge. Then twist left elbow over the right knee. Gently twist back again until facing forward, and stand up. Repeat with the other foot and arm.

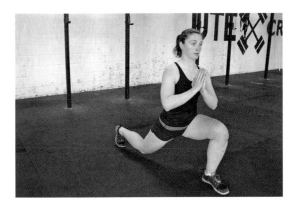 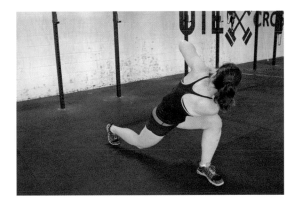

Shuffles: Start standing with feet together, with a slight bend in the knees. Step out with either foot so that your feet are about hip-width apart. Move laterally for about 20 meters, feel the explosiveness from your feet as you move across the room. For the more advanced athlete, start in a squatting position and stay in the low position across the room. Return to your starting position.

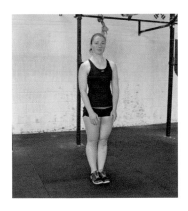 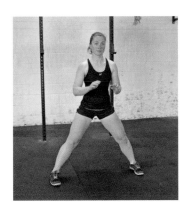 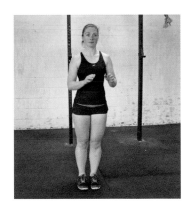

High Knees: Lightly jog picking up your knees as high as they can go, stretching out your legs as you move down the field.

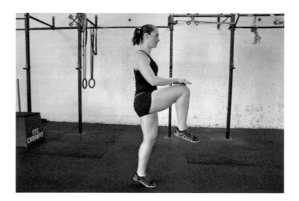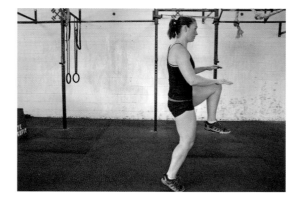

Butt Kickers: Lightly jog as before, this time kicking your feet back as you jog, trying to ultimately kick your butt with your foot.

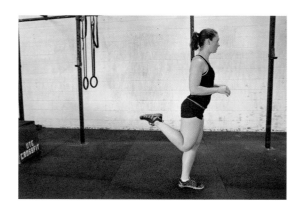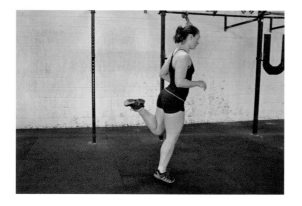

These are just a few of the exercises that can be used for active recovery. Whatever activity you choose, you should do something after your race to help get everything moving again and get you back to training for the next race!

CHAPTER 16
THE NEXT RACE

With your first race complete and your body back on the road to recovery as the bruises start to fade away, it is time to plan ahead to your next race. It is easy to get caught up in race fever[26] after completing your first obstacle race, and you just might find yourself seeking out more races late into the night. There is something about obstacle course racing that leaves you wanting more, wanting to try another race, waiting another chance to complete that failed obstacle. This is what keeps drawing people back to the sport week after week.

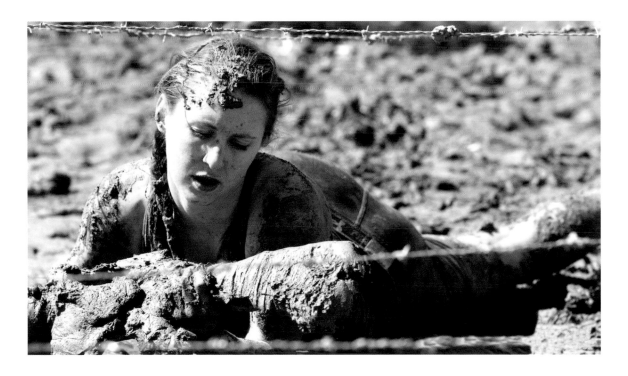

26 Race Fever is when you frantically start looking for every race around and available to you.

As you sit down to plot out your next race, it is important not to get too caught up in racing. With the explosion, of the sport, many urban areas have races almost every weekend within a few hours drive of any given town. A person could literally race every weekend of the year if they wanted. It is important to pick and choose when and where you race next. The first thing to consider is time off after your first race; you should give your body at least a month between races. This allows for the bruises and scrapes to fully heal and your body to recover completely. During the summer months, especially in cooler climates, races happen constantly and it is hard not want to race all the time. It takes a little bit of self-restraint to allow yourself to heal before heading off to the next event. At a minimum, you will want to give yourself three weeks (if you really can't hold out a whole month between races). If you do find yourself racing weekend after weekend you will need to listen to your body and take care of yourself as the season progresses. Many of the top athletes in the sport raced too much during the 2012 season only to find themselves fatigued and injured from over-racing going into 2013. At the end of the day it's about having fun, getting active and enjoying the experience. Only you can know what is too much for your body.

The second thing to consider is the distance race you would like to do. With your first race at around a 5K distance, you need to assess how your body handled it. Did you like the distance or would like to try something longer? Many event organizers now offer multiple distances for their participants; this way if you find an event you really like, you can try all the different distances. The Spartan Race and Superhero Scramble series both offer an additional medal if you complete all three available distances in a single season. This can be an added incentive to try the longer distances.

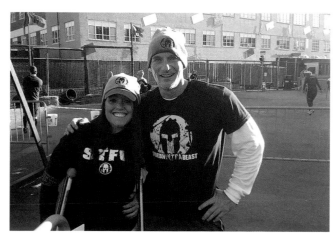

The important thing to remember when signing up for your next race is to find one that appeals to you. There are all sorts of races available today and each one has its own theme. There are zombie races, where people dressed up as zombies chase you. One new race is trying to play on all the elements. Others focus events around jungle, superhero, rebels, or other various themes. Pick a race that not only appeals to the distance you hope to run, but also the atmosphere you want to engage in.

With new races and challenges entering the market daily, you will surely be able to find another race that suits your wants and needs, now that you have had a taste of obstacle course racing. When planning out the rest of the year, you should focus on one race every month or so, depending on your location. It is important to keep a race/life balance as you continue in your obstacle course racing journey. It is easy to get sucked into it, wanting to try each race each weekend, until you soon find yourself traveling far distances to meet up with new friends and try new races. I personally fell victim to this cycle and have seen many friends in the sport follow suit. It is a fantastic way to see the country and spend time with newly formed friendships; however, it is important to save time for parties, friends' birthdays and other parts of life as well. There are a handful of athletes that make this sport their profession, but for the majority of people it is a weekend hobby and sport.

There is no doubt that you will find more races around you that spark your interest, maybe outside of the world of obstacle course racing as well. Many people find their own personal athlete inside them during their first obstacle course race, and months later find themselves signing up for a half marathon, marathon or trail race. Some will use an obstacle course race as the stepping-stone to other endurance-based sports. I remember one story of a woman who had never run before, trained for her first obstacle course race, finished, then looked for something else. About a year and a half later I received a message that she was now training for an Ironman triathlon. She had not been an athlete before that first race, but obstacle course racing was the spark she needed to pursue a healthy and active lifestyle.

Whether you find yourself dashing to find another obstacle course race, local 5K, half marathon, marathon, trail race or something in between, one thing is certain: you will want to keep yourself moving forward. You accomplished that first goal of completing the race, so now it is time to set a new goal and pursue the next challenge. Obstacle course racing shows you that you can accomplish anything. If you get Racing Fever, you will undoubtedly be back for more, searching out that next race to earn that coveted medal around your neck. Whatever you plan for your next race, the next time you step up to the starting line just know that you are stronger and even more capable than you once thought.

CHAPTER 17

INSIDER TIPS

Knowledge is the key to conquering most challenges in life, and the same is true with obstacle course racing. Among the many things worth knowing is how to mange the cost. Race entry fees can be expensive, and as you add more races to your calendar, the travel expenses also start to add up quickly. Here are a few tips and tricks to help make obstacle course racing more affordable.

Once you have tried out a few races and found a particular race organizer that you like more than the rest, check their website and see if they offer season passes. Many of the top race organizers are now offering these "bulk prices" for people looking to really jump into the sport of obstacle racing. The passes allow you to race anywhere in the country, some internationally as well; depending on your level of interest, it can take the price of racing down to a few dollars per race. Some organizations like Spartan Race give out a

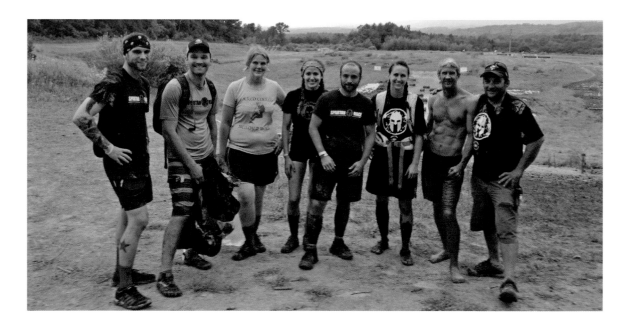

significant number of season passes each year depending on end-of-the-season rankings. If you catch the OCR bug and want to follow one event series, a season pass can be your ticket to expanding your geographic racing scope.

Volunteering is the single best way to earn yourself a free race, free parking, and a free t-shirt. Volunteering is the insider secret in obstacle course racing. Obstacle course races need a lot of volunteers, not only to help man registration, aid stations and obstacles, but to monitor penalty completion. This adds up to a lot of manpower and most race organizers are always clamoring for more help. Some race organizers choose to pay their "volunteers" for the day's worth of work, but increasingly race organizers are offering up other perks instead of a paycheck. Often those perks include that free entry to a later race, free parking, and free volunteer t-shirt. Volunteers also are given a meal while they are on course. Some races have even also added a designated volunteer heat for people who had volunteered all day, so they can race at the end of the day.

The most common way for volunteers to earn a free race is volunteering at a Saturday race, then running on Sunday. It is not explicitly offered that way, and in races that are only one-day events volunteers often race at the end of the day. Some of the most elite racers will even race on a Saturday then volunteer on a Sunday to earn another race at some future date.

Volunteering is also a fantastic way for many people to "get their feet wet" in obstacle course racing. I have met several people who had a race near their home and volunteered before becoming racers themselves. The volunteers get a first-hand look at the course. If you volunteer in the morning, you will likely see the competitive heats up close, so you will get a truly unique experience. Most event websites have a separate volunteer page, which details the exact type of perks they offer for helping out. Overall, volunteering can be a great way to help the growing sport, earn yourself a free race or two, and get an insider's view of the action.

Finally, the last option for earning a free race or other perks is to join a race organizer's "street team." Obstacle course racing was born of a grassroots sport, and continues to grow that way today. Most event organizers actively seek out people to help promote their brands and get more people signed up to race. These grassroots efforts can be as simple as, for example, the Superhero Scramble's promotion offering you free entry if you get three friends to sign up. Other event organizers give free entry to people who work expos, or hand out flyers at local gyms. Spartan Race has the most elaborate model for a street team, with perks ranging from a free entry up to a free trip to the world championships in Vermont at the end of the season. This model helps build the sport from the ground up and allows people who are passionate about obstacle course racing to spread the word about this burgeoning sport. Each event organizer is different and most have detailed their programs on the event website.

With a little bit of work and research, you might find yourself being able to travel around the country pursuing your new passion. There are many ways to get yourself to the starting line of the race; it all depends on your preferences. The most important thing is to read the event organizer's website; it is amazing how a few minutes online can save you hundreds of dollars in entry fees each year.

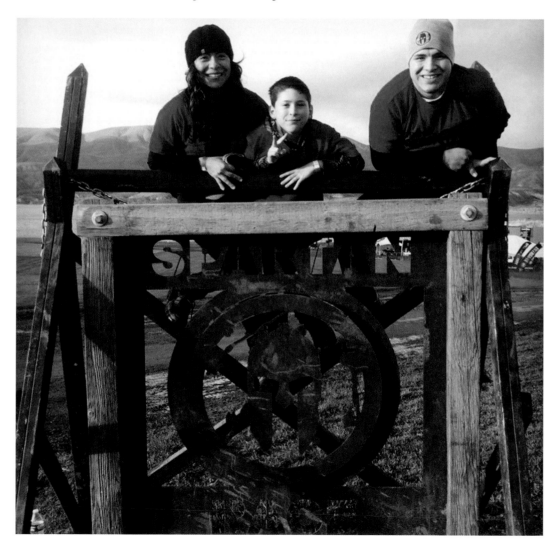

CHAPTER 18

CONTINUING THE JOURNEY

Over the course of this book you were introduced to the exciting new sport of obstacle course racing, learned the difference between mud runs and obstacle races, picked the perfect race for you to start with, gathered the tools on how to train and accomplish your first race, then walked all the way through race day and beyond. Hopefully this book has helped you get a taste for all things obstacle course racing. More importantly, I hope this book will be a stepping stone to a new you.

Obstacle course racing has a way of changing people. It is unique in that everyone can participate in it, and the fastest person and the slowest person complete the same course. It allows us to step out of the cubicle, out of the office, and away from the computer for a day. We get to challenge ourselves, get dirty, and feel the primal sense of living that is so often lost in our modern daily life. This is the beauty of obstacle course racing; it's raw, it's dirty, and it's above all something real.

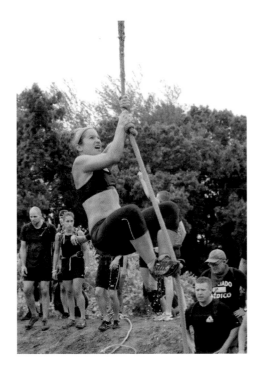

Over the years I have spoken to more and more people who tell the same story. They took on an obstacle course race for whatever initial reason and a few years later find themselves living active, healthier lifestyles because of taking the chance on that first race. Some never went back to another obstacle course race after the first, while others have made it their life's passion. Whatever the ultimate result, these people all have one thing in common: they took the chance and showed up, stepped onto the starting line and did the unknown.

Obstacle course racing has not only challenged me physically and mentally since I began my journey in 2010; It has also let me shine a mirror back at myself so that I could reexamine my life and where I was headed. Before obstacle course racing, I was just another ex-athlete who had gained about 20 pounds and enjoyed the mid-20s lifestyle. My first obstacle course race ignited my competitive fire again. It gave me the courage to see that I could make changes within myself. It propelled me to make drastic changes in life, leaving a career I had grown for almost a decade in order to start my own company, DirtinYourSkirt.com. It led me to realize that we can do whatever we truly want to and it's

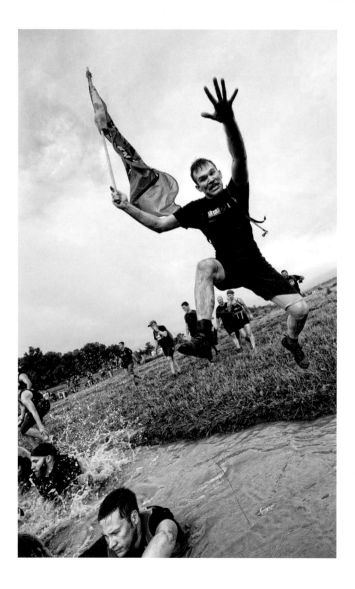

never too late to begin. It sounds silly that an hour in the mud and on the trails can have such profound reverberations into the rest of your life, but that is what obstacle course racing does.

It is your time to make your journey and use obstacle course racing as a piece in your puzzle. Maybe your goal is to someday run a marathon and this is the first step in that direction. The path is yours to take, and hopefully it is a muddy one. Enjoy the journey: it is your own.

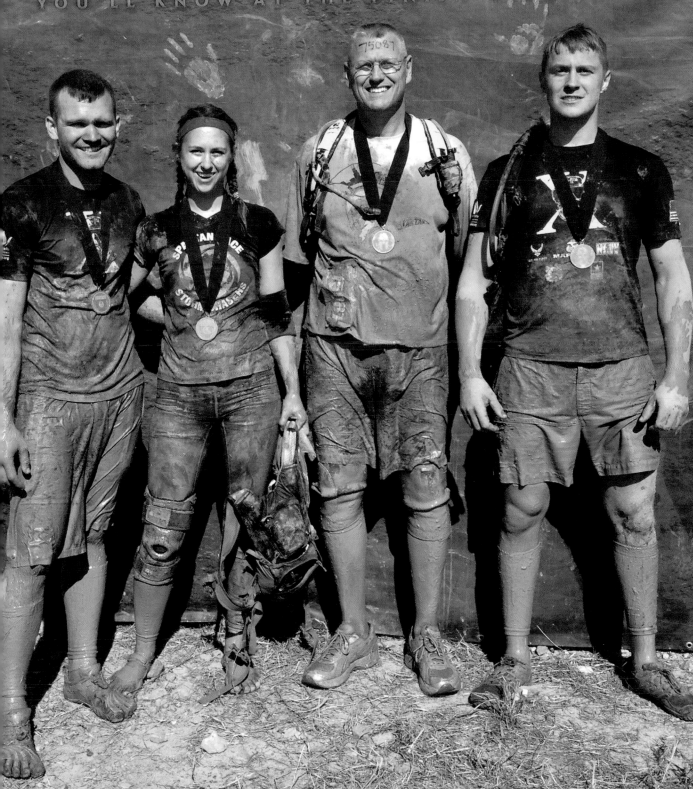

RACE DAY CHECKLIST

- Trail Shoes/Race Shoes
- Shorts/Capris
- Top
- Wicking Socks – NO COTTON
- Hydration Pack
- Sunscreen
- Small Towel
- Beach Towel
- Travel size biodegradable soap
- Post Race Clothing
- T-Shirt
- Shorts
- Sweatshirt/Fleece
- Underwear
- Hat
- Flip Flops or Extra Shoes
- Sunglasses
- Post Race Snacks & Hydration
- Cash
- Water
- Garbage Bag (for wet clothing)

APPENDIX 2
TRAINING LOG

Training logs are a key part of any training program. People who keep track of their training are more likely to keep at it and successfully meet goals. Logs are a great way to track progress and stay motivated. This training log can be adapted to almost any form of exercise and training. Below is an example of a training day.

When filling out the training log it is important to be honest with yourself and fill in the details. Use the "Workout Details" to describe the workout more fully. Try to be diligent about filling in all the boxes—even the "weather" box. Yes, the weather—it's an important factor to note, as you may find your intensity changes as the weather changes. Rate your workout honestly (you'll soon figure out what constitutes a good or bad workout for you). Finally, use the "workout feelings" section to describe what you were thinking, how your body felt, or something unique you saw or learned in the session. One more thing: don't skip the "sleep" box! Sleep is key to successful training and is often overlooked. Track your sleep patterns and you may find that your training intensity and sleep are more connected than you think!

If this log works for you as is, make copies of these pages and create a binder. If you like, take elements from it to create a log customized to your needs. One client added a column for checking off her daily water consumption, and another checks and logs his heart rate in the mornings. Whatever you do, make it your own, let it guide you and help you do your best.

Sample Entry:

MONDAY	DATE: *August 8*					Location: *Killington Mtn*	2nd Workout: N/A
Workout Time Start: *7.00AM*	Workout Time Finish						Workout Time: N/A
Workout Type: *RUN*	Run	Lift	Hike	Bike	Swim	Xfit	Details: *No second workout today*
Workout Details: *Hit the trails this morning for a long training run. Summited the peak and ran down while wearing a 10lb weight vest.*							
Distance: *8 Miles*	Time: *1:30*			Equipment			Daily Rate: 1 2 ③ 4 5
Weather: *Cloud/Dry*	Rate: *3* (1-worst, 5-Best)						Total Daily Miles: *8*
Workout Feelings: *Sluggish at first heading up the mountain. But once I got to the top it felt great to let the legs out and run down.*							Hours Sleep: *8*
							Other: *Had a great new recipe for chicken tonight.*

Your Training Journal

MONDAY	DATE:		Location:	2nd Workout
Workout Time Start:	Workout Time Finish			Workout Time:
Workout Type:	Run | Lift | Hike | Bike | Swim | Xfit			Details:
Workout Details:				
Distance:	Time:	Equipment		Daily Rate: 1 2 3 4 5
Weather:	Rate:			Total Daily Miles:
Workout Feelings:				Hours Sleep:
				Other:

TUESDAY	DATE:		Location:	2nd Workout
Workout Time Start:	Workout Time Finish			Workout Time:
Workout Type:	Run | Lift | Hike | Bike | Swim | Xfit			Details:
Workout Details:				
Distance:	Time:	Equipment		Daily Rate: 1 2 3 4 5
Weather:	Rate:			Total Daily Miles:
Workout Feelings:				Hours Sleep:
				Other:

WEDNESDAY	DATE:						Location:	2nd Workout
Workout Time Start:	Workout Time Finish							Workout Time:
Workout Type:	Run	Lift	Hike	Bike	Swim	Xfit		Details:
Workout Details:								
Distance:	Time:					Equipment		Daily Rate: 1 2 3 4 5
Weather:	Rate:							Total Daily Miles:
Workout Feelings:								Hours Sleep:
								Other:

THURSDAY	DATE:						Location:	2nd Workout
Workout Time Start:	Workout Time Finish							Workout Time:
Workout Type:	Run	Lift	Hike	Bike	Swim	Xfit		Details:
Workout Details:								
Distance:	Time:					Equipment		Daily Rate: 1 2 3 4 5
Weather:	Rate:							Total Daily Miles:
Workout Feelings:								Hours Sleep:
								Other:

FRIDAY	DATE:						Location:	2nd Workout
Workout Time Start:	Workout Time Finish							Workout Time:
Workout Type:	Run	Lift	Hike	Bike	Swim	Xfit		Details:
Workout Details:								
Distance:	Time:				Equipment			Daily Rate: 1 2 3 4 5
Weather:	Rate:							Total Daily Miles:
Workout Feelings:								Hours Sleep:
								Other:

SATURDAY	DATE:						Location:	2nd Workout
Workout Time Start:	Workout Time Finish							Workout Time:
Workout Type:	Run	Lift	Hike	Bike	Swim	Xfit		Details:
Workout Details:								
Distance:	Time:				Equipment			Daily Rate: 1 2 3 4 5
Weather:	Rate:							Total Daily Miles:
Workout Feelings:								Hours Sleep:
								Other:

SUNDAY	DATE:						Location:	2nd Workout
Workout Time Start:	Workout Time Finish							Workout Time:
Workout Type:	Run	Lift	Hike	Bike	Swim	Xfit		Details:
Workout Details:								
Distance:	Time:						Equipment	Daily Rate: 1 2 3 4 5
Weather:	Rate:							Total Daily Miles:
Workout Feelings:								Hours Sleep:
								Other:

WEEKLY OVERVIEW:	Dates:	Location:	
Overall:			
		TOTAL MILES/TIME:	
		RUN:	
		LIFT:	
		HIKE:	
		BIKE:	
		SWIM:	
		SKI:	
		Other:	
Total Hours Trained:		Details/Breakthoughs/Feelings:	
Total Hours Slept		Overall Rate: 1 2 3 4 5	
Injuries/Pain			

TURNING YOUR BACKYARD INTO A TRAINING CENTER

Sometimes going to the gym is not an option, and some local gyms don't have all the tools an obstacle course racer or mud runner needs to train properly for the next race, so more and more people are turning their backyards into training centers.

How to Build a Wall

One of the most versatile training tools you can build in your backyard is a wall. Legendary obstacle course racer Hobie Call was the first to add this tool to his backyard in 2011. Since then numerous people have built their own versions. The following is a modified version of his original wall and how to make it. This wall comes to about 7'6" tall.

Supplies:
 13 – 2"x6"x8' boards (pine works fine)
 10 – 2"x4"x8' boards (pine works fine)
 1 Box of 2½ inch screws (100+)
 2 – 10-foot long – 1¼ inch galvanized rigid steel pipes
 20 Metal connector plates
 5 Cans black spray paint (or color of choice)
 1 Electric saw
 1 Power drill (to screw in nails)

1. Cut 2x6's down to 7" long. This way you will have enough room on either side of the wall for the pull-up and muscle up bars.

2. Lay 2 – 2x4's across from each other on the ground. Starting from what will be the top of your wall, line up the 2x6's along the 2x4's. Insert the steel pipes at the appropriate heights for you (we like laying the first below the top board and the second below the forth board).

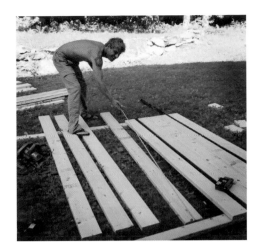

3. Screw the 2x6's into the 2x4's.

4. Measure the distance between the bottom of the last board and the bottom of the protruding 2x4. From two separate 2x4's cut a piece of wood to fit. (Set the remaining long pieces of 2x4 aside; these will form the bases of your trusses.) Screw the cut pieces flush, as shown.

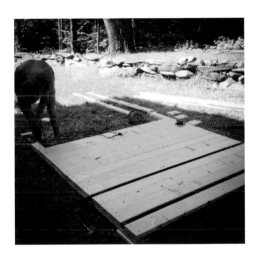

5. Reinforce your right and left sides by layering another 2x4 across your boards, in line with your original 2x4. In essence you are sandwiching your 2x6 boards between 2x4's. This adds extra security and rigidness to your wall.

6. Cut the 2x4's at an angle to form the side trusses. The angle and height will depend on where you place your muscle-up bar, so be sure to plan and measure accordingly. The bottom of the leg has to be flush with the bottom of your base board in order to lie level against the ground, so plan your bottom angles accordingly.

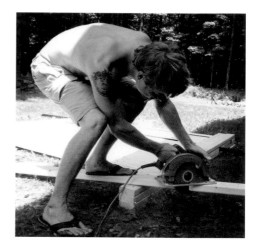

7. Screw the bottom of the legs to either end of the base. The tops of the legs should meet in a point. Screw those together or join using a connector plate if you want a more polished look (if you're feeling stuck, look ahead to the photos of the finished wall on p. 155).

8. Screw the base of your truss to the bottom end of the wall side, then screw the top of the truss into the wall side. (It should come just under the muscle up bar). Making your truss this way makes it easy to remove, in case your wall ever needs to be packed flat for moving and storing.

9. Once the wall is complete, you can add 2x4 wood (excess from the truss construction) to create a kicker or helper step. This is used in many races and also is nice when going over the wall multiple times. Place the board (should be about 6 inches long) over the third from bottom board. Screw into the 2x6 on the wall with 3-4 screws.

10. Spray paint the wall. The paint helps weatherize it and adds a nice clean look. We got fancy and added the Dirt in Your Skirt Logo to ours. (p. 155.)

Once your wall is built there are hundreds of ways to use it in your training. This is one of our favorite workouts using the wall. All you need is your wall and a sandbag.

5 sets each set includes:
1. Throw sandbag over wall
2. Climb over wall
3. Throw sandbag back over wall
4. Climb under wall

Repeat 10 times...

Modifications:

More and more people are also coupling their wall with a spear and spear-throwing target. Below are instructions how to build a spear and target to attach to your wall. People commonly ask how much distance should be between you and the target. The answer is that it varies by race, so if you build a spear and target you should practice at various distances.

How to Build a Basic Spear:

Supplies:
60" bow rake handle replacement
10" or 12" ¼ inch galvanized spike
Gorilla Glue
Grinder

1. Cut the top of the spike off. The spike should fit perfectly into the tip of the rake replacement. (Test in store to make sure it's the right spike.)

2. Place a small amount of glue in the hole of the handle. Insert the spike. Allow to dry for 12-24 hours.

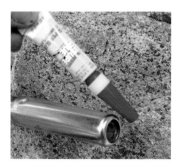 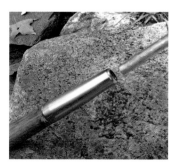

3. To see fancier versions of the spear go to www.dirtinyourskirt.com for the Spartan Race - Race Director approved deluxe spear kit.

How to build a Target:

Supplies:
1 – Bail of hay
1 – 3' x 24' Burlap roll
1 - 3/8" Diamond Braid Poly Rope (anything over 20 feet will do)
2 – X-Large carabiners

1. Wrap hay in burlap. Covering the hay in burlap will help keep the bail together after repeated throws.

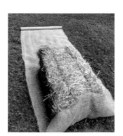

2. Cut two lengths of rope and tie loops on each end.

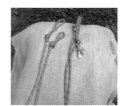

3. Wrap rope vertically around bail and through loops.

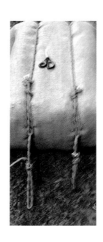

4. Cut two more lengths of rope and wrap rope horizontally around vertical rope.

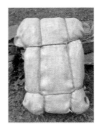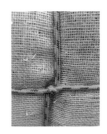

5. Tuck burlap and tie off rope. Tuck last sections in and spray paint a target (optional).

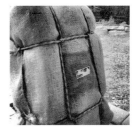

6. Clip carabiner to rope and hang off pull-up bar on your wall.

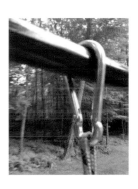

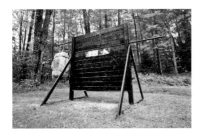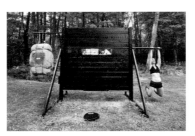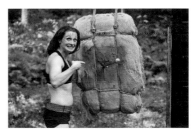

This is your finished practice wall, complete with target.

Other common training tools: Ropes and tires. Depending on your location these may also be added to your personal backyard playground.

APPENDIX 4
GOAL SETTING

As briefly discussed in Chapter 7 goal setting is an integral part of success in any training program. Not setting goals in your fitness and health is like driving down a road with no known destination; you can keep going but if you don't have a destination, or plan stops along the way, you will find yourself aimlessly wandering forever. Below are a few steps to help you organize your goals, and a goal sheet to for you to write them down and hold yourself accountable.

1. Goals must be YOUR goals. Set goals you want to achieve.
2. Goals must be specific, measurable, and observable.
3. Set a timeline – a beginning of the goal and an end point.
4. Set difficult but attainable goals.
5. Goals should be easy to monitor for process. There are three types of goals process, performance and outcome. A balanced goal sheet should include all three.
6. Incorporate micro-goals (short term) into a long-term program. Set daily goals in each training session to help achieve the long term.
7. Set positive goals, and avoid the negative (e.g. positive – complete monkey bars; negative – fail fewer obstacles).
8. Share your goals and hold yourself accountable.
9. Seek the support of others to help you achieve your goals.
10. Be flexible when goals change – it's a process, and goals often need to be adjusted.

Use "SMARTS" When Goal Setting

Time-management consultant Hyrum W. Smith[1] created this acronym to help people achieve effective goal setting. These can all be easily applied to sport as well as life. Keep "SMARTS" in mind when you fill out your goal-setting sheet.

---

1   Smith H. 1995. *10 Natural Laws of Successful Time and Life Management*. Warner Books Inc. New York, NY.

S = Specific – "place higher" or "run faster" are vague, instead "place in top 15" or "finish the race in under and hour."

M = Measurable – Quantify goals. Set times and number, for example, 100 sit-ups in under 3 minutes.

A = Action-Oriented – Goals should guide actions.

R = Realistic – Make goals attainable but challenging.

T = Timely – Have a time frame.

S = Self-Determined – It's your training, so the goals need to be meaningful to you.

Goal Sheet

"Do not let what you can't do interfere with what you can do."   —John Wooden

Name: _____ Today's Date: _____

Start Date: _____ Target Date: _____

One sport based-goal for the season/year:

What are three steps you are going to take to achieve that goal?

Goal Pyramid: (Fill the pyramid)   Long Term (Dream) Goal

Intermediate Goal

Short Term Goal

Immediate (Process) Goals – The Daily How

Where are two places you will list your goal? (Place it where you can see it each day.)
Who are two people who will help you reach your goal? (Give them your goal sheet.)
Write FIVE goals YOU REALLY want to accomplish this year (make sure to apply SMARTS):

1. Sport-Based Goal – Competition
2. Sport-Based Goal - Training
3. Life-Based Goal
4. Work-Based Goal
5. Other Goal (Sport, Life, Work, Relationship, etc…)

We are often our own worst enemy and spend much of our time fighting not against competitors, but against ourselves. The exercise below is a tool to help raise your self-awareness, adapted from the USFSA, used by elite level-athletes. Below list POSTITIVE attributes you hold to complete each of the sentences; you may use examples both in and out of sport.

Self Confidence Exercise
Something I do well during an obstacle course race or mud run: ....

Something I do even better in obstacle course racing or mud runs is: ....

My greatest strength as an athlete is: ....

I am proud that I: ....

My greatest strength is: ....

I have the power to: ....

I was able to decide to: ....

I am not afraid to: ....

Something that I can do now that I couldn't last year: ....

I have accomplished: ....

If I want to, I can: ....

My greatest achievement is: ....

Spend time developing this list, refer back to it monthly, make changes, you can push boundaries and create new experiences. Instead of focusing on what you can't do focus on the can, and build off of it. Once you begin to focus on the positive, the things that once seemed difficult look a little less daunting next time you try them.

Index

Photo Credits:

The Tuttle Story
"Books to Span the East and West"

Many people are surprised to learn that the world's largest publisher of books on Asia had its humble beginnings in the tiny American state of Vermont. The company's founder, Charles E. Tuttle, belonged to a New England family steeped in publishing.

Immediately after WW II, Tuttle served in Tokyo under General Douglas MacArthur and was tasked with reviving the Japanese publishing industry. He later founded the Charles E. Tuttle Publishing Company, which thrives today as one of the world's leading independent publishers.

Though a westerner, Tuttle was hugely instrumental in bringing a knowledge of Japan and Asia to a world hungry for information about the East. By the time of his death in 1993, Tuttle had published over 6,000 books on Asian culture, history and art—a legacy honored by the Japanese emperor with the "Order of the Sacred Treasure," the highest tribute Japan can bestow upon a non-Japanese.

With a backlist of 1,500 titles, Tuttle Publishing is more active today than at any time in its past—inspired by Charles Tuttle's core mission to publish fine books to span the East and West and provide a greater understanding of each.